Juicing for vitality and wellness

The essential guide to health and nutrition.

By

Walter . E . Mark

Copyright page

Copyright © 2024 Walter. E . Mark.

 All rights reserved.

No part of this book may be reproduced, distributed, or transmitted in any form or by any means, including photocopying, recording, or other electronic or mechanical methods, without the prior written permission of the publisher, except in the case of brief quotations embodied in critical reviews .

Table of content

Chapter 1

Introduction: Juicing - The Elixir of Life

In the heart of nature's bounty lies the secret to vitality and wellness—a secret as simple as the fruits and vegetables that adorn our tables. This book is an ode to the power of juicing, a practice that transforms these humble ingredients into elixirs of health. As we stand at the threshold of 2024, the world is awakening to the profound benefits that juicing has to offer. It's not just a trend; it's a lifestyle, a remedy, and a celebration of life's purest flavors.

The Journey of Juicing

Our journey begins with the roots of juicing, tracing back to ancient civilizations where the extraction of juice was a means to harness the medicinal properties of plants. Through the ages, this art has evolved, transcending borders and cultures, to become a cornerstone of health regimens around the globe. Today, juicing is not just about sustenance; it's about thriving. It's a testament to the fact that the most potent remedies are often the most natural ones.

The Science of Synergy

Juicing is the alchemy of converting whole fruits and vegetables into a form that our bodies can absorb more readily. It's a synergy of science and nature, where each sip delivers a concentrated dose of vitamins, minerals, enzymes, and phytonutrients. These components work in harmony to fortify our bodies, boost our immune systems, and rejuvenate our cells. In this book, we delve into the scientific underpinnings that make juicing a powerful tool for health and healing.

A Palette of Nutrients

Imagine a palette where kale's deep greens, beetroot's vibrant reds, and the sunny hues of citrus come together to create a masterpiece of nutrition. Juicing allows us to paint with these colors, crafting concoctions that please the palate while nourishing the body. We'll explore the nutritional profiles of various produce and how they contribute to our health, providing you with the knowledge to create your own nutrient-dense juices.

Juicing for the Soul

But juicing is more than a physical health practice; it's a ritual that nourishes the soul. It's a moment of mindfulness in our day, a creative outlet, and a connection to the food we consume. This book will guide you through the sensory experience of juicing—the sounds, the smells, and the flavors that make it a meditative and gratifying practice.

Your Personal Health Ally

Whether you're seeking to address specific health concerns, enhance your energy levels, or embark on a journey of detoxification, this book will serve as your personal health ally. We'll introduce you to recipes designed for various health goals and teach you how to tailor your juicing practice to your unique needs.

The Juicing Community

As you turn the pages of this book, you're joining a community of like-minded individuals who have embraced juicing as a path to wellness. We'll share stories of transformation, tips from experts, and insights from fellow juicing enthusiasts. Together, we'll celebrate the victories and navigate the challenges on the road to optimal health.

Embarking on Your Juicing Adventure

This book is your map to the world of juicing. Each chapter is a step on the path, leading you deeper into the practice and closer to the health you desire. We invite you to approach this journey with curiosity and an open heart, ready to discover the wonders that juicing has in store for you.

As you embark on this adventure, remember that every choice you make at the juicer is a step toward a more vibrant, energetic, and healthy life. So let's begin this transformative journey together, one juice at a time.

Chapter 2

Juicing basics

Juicing is a transformative practice that has been embraced by cultures around the world for its health benefits and the pure enjoyment it brings. It's a process that involves extracting the liquid part of fruits and vegetables, leaving behind the fiber, and consuming a nutrient-dense beverage that can be easily absorbed by the body. This simple yet profound act of drinking juice allows individuals to consume a higher volume of fruits and vegetables than they would typically eat, providing a convenient way to increase one's intake of essential vitamins, minerals, and antioxidants.

The Essence of Juicing

At its core, juicing is about breaking down fresh produce to release the vital nutrients contained within. When we juice, we're able to access the rich spectrum of nutrients that are often locked away in the fibers of fruits and vegetables. These nutrients include a variety of vitamins, such as vitamin C and vitamin K, essential minerals like potassium and magnesium, enzymes that aid digestion, and a host of phytonutrients that offer numerous health benefits.

The Benefits of Juicing

The benefits of juicing are manifold. For starters, it can enhance nutrient absorption because the body doesn't have to work as hard to break down the fiber of the whole fruit or vegetable. This is particularly beneficial for those with a compromised digestive system or for elderly individuals who may have difficulty digesting fiber-rich foods. Moreover, juicing can help increase your intake of antioxidants, which play a crucial role in combating oxidative stress and inflammation in the body.

Juicing vs. Blending

It's important to distinguish between juicing and blending. While both are excellent ways to consume fruits and vegetables, they serve different purposes. Blending retains the fiber, resulting in a thicker drink like a smoothie, which can aid in digestion and help you feel full. Juicing, on the other hand, removes most of the fiber, resulting in a thinner, more concentrated liquid that allows for quicker absorption of nutrients.

Types of Juicers

The type of juicer you choose can also impact the quality of your juice. Centrifugal juicers are popular for their speed and convenience, but they can introduce heat and oxidation, which may reduce the nutrient content of the juice. Masticating juicers, also known as cold-press juicers, operate at a slower speed, minimizing heat and preserving more of the delicate enzymes and nutrients. Triturating juicers, with their twin gears, offer the highest yield and nutrient retention but come at a higher cost and require more effort to use.

The Role of Fiber

While juicing removes most of the fiber, it's worth noting that the resulting beverage still contains soluble fiber. Soluble fiber dissolves in water and can help to lower glucose levels and blood cholesterol. The insoluble fiber, which is left behind, aids in moving food through the digestive system and is beneficial for bowel health. Therefore, it's recommended to maintain a balance between juicing and consuming whole fruits and vegetables to ensure you're getting enough fiber in your diet.

Juicing for Health Conditions

Juicing can be particularly beneficial for individuals with specific health conditions. For example, juices rich in ginger and turmeric can have anti-inflammatory effects, which may benefit those with conditions like arthritis. Beetroot juice is known for its ability to lower blood pressure and enhance athletic performance due to its nitrate content. Green juices, packed with leafy greens like kale and spinach, are high in chlorophyll and can support detoxification processes in the body.

Customizing Your Juice

One of the joys of juicing is the ability to customize your concoctions to suit your taste preferences and nutritional needs. You can create a juice that targets your health goals, whether it's boosting immunity with citrus fruits, enhancing skin health with cucumber and aloe vera, or increasing energy levels with a blend of green vegetables and apples.

Juicing as a Lifestyle

Adopting juicing as part of your lifestyle can lead to positive changes in your overall health and well-being. It encourages you to make conscious choices about what you put into your body and can be a stepping stone to adopting other healthy habits. Many people find that starting their day with a fresh juice sets a healthful tone for the rest of the day, leading to better food choices and a more active lifestyle.

Juicing is a powerful tool in the pursuit of health and vitality. It allows us to consume a high concentration of nutrients in an easily digestible form, supports various health conditions, and can be customized to fit individual needs. Whether you're a seasoned juicer or just beginning your journey, the world of juicing offers a delicious and nutritious way to enhance your health and enjoy the natural goodness of fruits and vegetables.

This introduction to juicing provides a comprehensive overview of the practice, its benefits, and how it can be integrated into a healthy lifestyle. As you delve deeper into the world of juicing, you'll discover the many ways in which this simple practice can have a profound impact on your health and well-being.

Types of juicers

Juicing has become a popular way to consume essential nutrients from fruits and vegetables quickly and deliciously. The cornerstone of this practice is the juicer itself, a device designed to extract juice from produce efficiently. Understanding the different types of juicers is crucial for anyone looking to start or enhance their juicing journey. Each type of juicer comes with its own set of features, benefits, and considerations. Here, we delve into the world of juicers, exploring the various types available on the market and how they can cater to different juicing preferences and lifestyles.

Centrifugal Juicers: The Speedy Solution

Centrifugal juicers are perhaps the most common type found in households due to their speed and convenience. These juicers use a fast-spinning metal blade that cuts the fruits and vegetables and spins them at high speed to separate the juice from the pulp through centrifugal force. The juice is then strained through a mesh filter and collected into a container, while the pulp is discarded separately.

Pros:

- Quick Juicing: Ideal for busy individuals who want to make juice in a hurry.

- Ease of Use: Generally user-friendly with simple assembly and operation.

- Cost-Effective: Often more affordable than other types of juicers.

Cons:

- Oxidation: The high speed generates heat, which can cause oxidation, potentially reducing the nutritional content.

- Noise: Tend to be louder than other types of juicers.

- Juice Quality: May not extract as much juice from leafy greens and soft fruits.

Masticating Juicers: The Nutrient Preservers

Masticating juicers, also known as cold press or slow juicers, operate by crushing and pressing the produce to extract juice. They use a single auger that slowly rotates to crush the fruit or vegetable against a stainless steel mesh screen. This slow process minimizes heat and oxidation, preserving more nutrients and enzymes in the juice.

Pros:

- Higher Nutrient Retention: The slow juicing process helps retain more vitamins, minerals, and enzymes.

- Versatility: Can handle a wide variety of produce, including leafy greens and wheatgrass.

- Quiet Operation: Operates more quietly compared to centrifugal juicers.

Cons:

- Slower Juicing Time: Not as fast as centrifugal juicers, requiring more patience.

- Price: Generally more expensive than centrifugal models.

- Size and Weight: Tend to be heavier and take up more counter space.

Triturating Juicers: The Maximum Yield Experts

Triturating juicers, or twin gear juicers, are the top-of-the-line when it comes to juicing. They have two interlocking gears that rotate inward and crush everything between them. The produce is ground to a fine pulp, and the juice is squeezed out through a screen. This process is highly efficient, producing a very dry pulp and extracting the maximum amount of juice and nutrients.

Pros:

- Optimal Extraction: Provides the highest yield and nutrient extraction among juicer types.

- Versatility: Excellent for juicing a wide range of produce, including tough, fibrous vegetables and leafy greens.

- Low Oxidation: The slow turning of the gears minimizes heat and oxidation.

Cons:

- Cost: These are typically the most expensive juicers on the market.

- Complexity: Can be more challenging to assemble, operate, and clean.

- Time-Consuming: The juicing process is slower, requiring more preparation time.

Hydraulic Press Juicers: The Pressure Powerhouses

Hydraulic press juicers use tremendous pressure to extract juice. The produce is first ground into a pulp, which is then placed into a cloth bag or directly onto a press. The hydraulic press then exerts force to squeeze out every last drop of juice. This method is known for producing extremely high-quality juice with minimal oxidation.

Pros:

- Quality Juice: Yields juice with the highest nutritional quality and longest shelf life.

- Efficiency: Extracts the most juice possible, leaving an extremely dry pulp.

- Gentle Process: The absence of heat and air keeps the juice's enzymes and nutrients intact.

Cons:

- High Price Point: Among the most expensive juicers available.

- Manual Labor: Some models require manual effort to press the juice.

- Cleaning and Maintenance: Can be more labor-intensive to clean and maintain.

Manual Juicers: The Simple Classics

Manual juicers are hand-operated and require no electricity. They range from simple citrus reamers to more complex lever-action presses. These juicers are perfect for those who juice occasionally or want to have control over the juicing process.

Pros:

- Portability: No need for electricity, making them ideal for travel or outdoor use.

- Ease of Cleaning: Fewer parts and no electrical components make them easy to clean.

- Affordability: Generally the most cost-effective option.

Cons:

- Physical Effort: Requires manual force to extract juice.

- Limited Use: Best suited for citrus fruits and may not be effective for other types of produce.

- Time-Consuming: Not as efficient as electric juicers for making larger quantities of juice.

Choosing the Right Juicer

Selecting the right juicer comes down to personal preference, budget, and intended use. If speed and convenience are your priorities, a centrifugal juicer might be the best choice. For those who prioritize nutritional content and are willing to invest more time and money, masticating or triturating juicers are excellent options. Hydraulic press juicers offer the highest quality juice, while manual juicers appeal to those seeking simplicity and portability.

The type of juicer you choose will significantly impact your juicing experience. By understanding the different types of juicers and their respective pros and cons, you can make an informed decision that aligns with your lifestyle and juicing goals. Whether you're a health enthusiast, a busy professional, or someone who enjoys the occasional fresh juice, there's a juicer out there that's perfect for you.

Selecting your produce

Selecting the right produce for juicing is a critical step in the process of creating nutritious and delicious juices. The quality, freshness, and variety of the fruits and vegetables you choose will directly impact the taste and health benefits of your juice. Here's an in-depth guide to help you make the best choices for your juicing needs.

Understanding Produce Quality

The foundation of good juice starts with high-quality produce. When selecting fruits and vegetables for juicing, consider the following factors:

- Freshness: Fresh produce not only tastes better but also contains the highest level of nutrients. Look for fruits and vegetables that are firm, vibrant in color, and free from bruises or blemishes.

- Ripeness: Ripe produce yields more juice and provides a sweeter, more robust flavor. Fruits should be slightly soft to the touch, while vegetables should be firm and not wilted.

- Organic vs. Conventional: Organic produce is grown without synthetic pesticides and fertilizers, making it a healthier choice for juicing. If organic options are not available or affordable, ensure to wash conventional produce thoroughly.

- Seasonality: Seasonal fruits and vegetables are often fresher and more flavorful. They are also typically more affordable and environmentally friendly since they don't require long-distance transportation.

Nutritional Considerations

When juicing, it's essential to consider the nutritional content of the produce you select:

- Variety: Incorporate a wide range of fruits and vegetables to ensure a diverse intake of vitamins, minerals, and antioxidants. Each color represents different nutrients, so aim for a rainbow of produce in your juices.

- Greens: Leafy greens like kale, spinach, and Swiss chard are packed with chlorophyll, vitamins, and minerals. They are a staple in many juice recipes for their health benefits.

- Fruits: While fruits add sweetness and flavor, they also contain natural sugars. Balance fruit with vegetables to avoid a sugar spike.

- Herbs and Spices: Don't forget to add herbs like parsley, cilantro, or mint, and spices like ginger or turmeric for additional health benefits and flavor complexity.

The taste of your juice is just as important as its nutritional value. Consider the following when selecting produce:

- Sweet: Apples, pears, and carrots can add natural sweetness to your juice.

- Tart: Citrus fruits like lemons, limes, and grapefruits can provide a refreshing tartness.

- Earthy: Beets and sweet potatoes offer an earthy depth to juice blends.

- Spicy: A small piece of ginger or a dash of cayenne pepper can add a spicy kick to your juice.

Juicing Different Types of Produce

Different fruits and vegetables require different juicing approaches:

- Leafy Greens: Roll or bunch up leafy greens before juicing to maximize yield.

- Soft Fruits: Soft fruits like berries and peaches may need to be juiced with harder produce to push them through the juicer.

- Hard Vegetables: Hard vegetables like carrots and beets should be cut into smaller pieces to prevent strain on the juicer.

Storing Your Produce

Proper storage can extend the freshness of your produce:

- Refrigeration: Most fruits and vegetables should be stored in the refrigerator to maintain freshness.

- Countertop: Some fruits, like bananas and avocados, ripen best at room temperature.

- Separation: Certain fruits emit ethylene gas, which can cause other produce to ripen prematurely. Store these separately.

Prepping for Juicing

Before juicing, take the time to properly prepare your produce:

- Washing: Use a produce wash or a mixture of water and vinegar to clean fruits and vegetables thoroughly.

- Peeling: Some fruits and vegetables should be peeled to remove bitter skins or inedible parts.

- Chopping: Cut produce into pieces that will fit easily into your juicer's feed chute.

Sourcing Your Produce

Where you get your produce can also make a difference:

- Farmers' Markets: Local farmers' markets are excellent sources of fresh, seasonal produce.

- Community-Supported Agriculture (CSA): Joining a CSA can provide you with a regular supply of fresh produce directly from local farms.

- Grocery Stores: When shopping at grocery stores, look for produce that is labeled as locally grown or organic.

Selecting the right produce for juicing is a multifaceted process that involves considering quality, nutrition, flavor, and preparation. By taking the time to choose the best fruits and vegetables for your juices, you'll not only enjoy tastier beverages but also reap the maximum health benefits. Remember, the key to great juicing starts with great produce, so choose wisely and juice happily!

Juicing techniques

Juicing techniques are the cornerstone of creating delicious and nutritious juices. Whether you're a beginner or an experienced juicer, understanding the nuances of these techniques can greatly enhance the quality of your juice. Here's an in-depth exploration of juicing techniques that will help you master the art of juicing.

The Art of Juicing: Techniques for Maximizing Flavor and Nutrition

Juicing is not just about throwing fruits and vegetables into a machine; it's about understanding how to extract the maximum amount of nutrients and flavor from your produce. Here are some advanced techniques to consider:

1. Preparation: Proper preparation of produce is essential. Wash all fruits and vegetables thoroughly to remove dirt and pesticides. Organic produce is preferred to reduce the intake of harmful chemicals. For harder vegetables like carrots and beets, peeling may be necessary to avoid bitter flavors. Leafy greens should be washed and then dried to prevent dilution of flavor.

2. Layering: When adding produce to the juicer, layer soft and hard ingredients. Start with softer items like citrus and tomatoes, which can sometimes clog the juicer if not pushed through by harder produce like apples and carrots. This technique ensures a consistent flow and prevents wastage.

3. Combining Flavors: Understanding flavor profiles is crucial. Sweet fruits can balance the bitterness of greens, while citrus can add a refreshing zing. Experiment with different combinations to find what pleases your palate while also providing a variety of nutrients.

4. Juicing Order: The order in which you juice ingredients can affect the final taste. Juice leafy greens first, as they yield less liquid and can be pushed through by juicier fruits and vegetables. Finish with high-yield produce like cucumbers or oranges to flush through any remaining bits.

5. Pulp Recycling: The pulp produced during juicing is rich in fiber and can be used in various recipes, from veggie burgers to soups and broths. This not only reduces waste but also ensures you benefit from the whole produce.

6. Temperature: The temperature of your produce can impact the juice's flavor and nutrient content. Cold produce can make the juice more refreshing and can also help to preserve enzymes and vitamins that are sensitive to heat.

7. Speed Settings: If your juicer has multiple speed settings, use them strategically. Slow speeds are better for leafy greens and soft fruits, which can get shredded too finely at high speeds, while harder produce benefits from faster speeds.

8. Timing: Drink juice immediately after making it to benefit from the maximum amount of nutrients before they degrade. If you must store it, use an airtight container and refrigerate to slow down nutrient loss.

9. Cleaning: Clean your juicer immediately after use. Dried pulp is harder to remove and can harbor bacteria. Disassemble the juicer completely and use brushes to clean screens and nooks.

10. Maintenance: Regularly check your juicer for signs of wear and tear, especially on blades and filters. Sharp blades are essential for efficient juicing and nutrient extraction.

11. Advanced Techniques: For those looking to take their juicing to the next level, consider advanced techniques such as:

   - Juice Pairing: Similar to wine pairing, juice pairing involves matching the right juice with meals to enhance the dining experience.

   - Juice Fasting: A juice fast involves consuming only juice for a set period to detoxify the body and reset the digestive system.

   - Therapeutic Juicing: This involves creating juice recipes targeted at specific health issues, such as inflammation or digestive problems.

12. Education: Continuously educate yourself on the health benefits of different produce and stay updated on new juicing trends and research. This knowledge will allow you to create juices that are not only tasty but also tailored to your health needs.

By mastering these juicing techniques, you can ensure that every glass of juice is a delightful blend of flavors and nutrients. Remember, juicing is a journey, and the more you practice, the better your results will be. So, embrace the process, experiment with new ingredients, and enjoy the health benefits that come with it.

Cleaning and Mantenance

Maintaining and cleaning your juicer is essential to ensure its longevity, efficiency, and the quality of juice it produces. Proper care prevents the buildup of residue and bacteria, which can affect the taste of your juice and potentially pose health risks. Here's a comprehensive guide to keeping your juicer in top condition.

Daily Cleaning Routine

A daily cleaning routine is vital for any juicer. After each use, disassemble the juicer to clean all parts that come into contact with food. This includes the feed chute, pulp container, juice jug, and any filters or blades. Use warm, soapy water and a soft brush or sponge to gently scrub away pulp and residue. For tough spots, a nylon brush can be effective, especially for cleaning mesh screens and filters.

Deep Cleaning

At least once a week, perform a deep cleaning of your juicer. Soak removable parts in a mixture of water and vinegar or a specialized cleaning solution to help dissolve any buildup and sanitize the components. Use a small brush or an old toothbrush to clean hard-to-reach areas and remove any remaining debris. Rinse all parts thoroughly with warm water and allow them to air dry completely before reassembling the juicer.

Handling Clogs and Stains

If your juicer becomes clogged, do not attempt to force it to continue operating. Turn off the machine, unplug it, and disassemble it to locate and remove the blockage. For stains, especially from colorful produce like beets and carrots, create a paste with baking soda and water and apply it to the stained areas. Let it sit for a few minutes before scrubbing and rinsing.

Blade and Filter Maintenance

The blades and filters are crucial for the juicer's performance. Dull blades can tear produce rather than cut cleanly, which can affect the quality of the juice and cause the motor to work harder. Sharpen the blades as needed, and replace them if they become too worn. Filters should be checked regularly for any tears or damage and replaced if necessary to ensure the finest quality juice.

Motor and Electrical Care

The motor is the heart of your juicer, and taking care of it is essential. Avoid overloading the juicer, as this can strain the motor and reduce its lifespan. If your juicer starts to sound strained or overheats, turn it off and let it cool down before continuing. Keep the motor base clean by wiping it with a damp cloth, but never immerse it in water or any other liquid.

Lubrication

Some juicers have parts that require lubrication to function smoothly. Consult your juicer's manual to determine if any components need lubrication and use only food-grade lubricants. Apply lubricant sparingly to avoid attracting dust and pulp, which can gum up the moving parts.

Storage

When not in use, store your juicer in a clean, dry place. If you're storing it assembled, ensure all parts are dry to prevent mold and mildew growth. If you're storing it disassembled, keep all parts together in a container or bag to prevent loss or damage.

Regular Inspections

Regularly inspect your juicer for signs of wear and tear. Check for cracks, loose components, or any changes in performance. Addressing issues early can prevent more significant problems down the line and can save you time and money on repairs.

Professional Servicing

For more complex issues or regular maintenance checks, consider professional servicing. Some manufacturers offer servicing and part replacement as part of their offerings. Professional servicing can ensure that your juicer is in optimal condition and can help extend its lifespan.

User Manual Guidance

Always refer to your juicer's user manual for specific instructions on cleaning and maintenance. The manual will provide guidance tailored to your model, including how to safely disassemble and reassemble the juicer, recommended cleaning products, and a maintenance schedule.

Cleaning and maintaining your juicer may seem like a chore, but it's a small price to pay for the benefits of fresh, healthy juice. A well-maintained juicer will serve you for many years, providing delicious and nutritious juices that can enhance your health and well-being. By following these guidelines, you'll ensure that your juicer remains a reliable and valuable part of your daily routine.

Chapter 3

Juicing for health

Juicing for detoxification

Juicing for detoxification is a concept that has gained popularity in the wellness community, with many people turning to juice cleanses as a means to purportedly eliminate toxins from the body, reset their digestive system, and promote overall health. However, it's essential to approach this topic with a critical eye, as the scientific evidence supporting the efficacy of juice cleanses for detoxification is limited. Below is an in-depth exploration of the subject.

Understanding Detoxification

Detoxification is a natural process carried out by the body, primarily by the liver and kidneys, to remove waste products and harmful substances. These organs work continuously to filter the blood, break down toxins, and excrete them through urine, feces, and sweat. The concept of "detoxing" through diet, particularly juicing, is based on the belief that certain foods can enhance these natural processes or help the body "flush out" toxins more effectively.

The Appeal of Juice Cleanses

Juice cleanses typically involve consuming only fruit and vegetable juices for a set period, ranging from a day to several weeks. Proponents claim that this practice can lead to various health benefits, including improved digestion, clearer skin, increased energy levels, and even weight loss. The idea is that by eliminating solid foods and consuming only juices, the digestive system is given a break from processing complex foods, allowing it to focus on healing and rejuvenation.

Potential Benefits of Juicing for Detoxification

- Nutrient Intake: Juices are rich in vitamins, minerals, and phytonutrients, providing a concentrated source of nutrition. For example, they can be high in vitamin C, potassium, and antioxidants, which play roles in immune function and cellular protection.

- Hydration: Juicing increases fluid intake, which can support kidney function and help in the elimination of water-soluble toxins.

- Digestive Rest: A temporary shift to an all-liquid diet may give the digestive system a brief respite from breaking down solid foods, potentially aiding in gut health recovery.

The Science Behind Juicing for Detoxification

Despite the claims, there is a lack of robust scientific evidence to support the idea that juice cleanses can detoxify the body. The liver and kidneys are highly efficient at filtering and eliminating toxins without the need for special diets. Moreover, many of the benefits attributed to juice cleanses, such as weight loss and improved skin condition, can often be attributed to the caloric restriction and increased hydration associated with these regimens, rather than the detoxification process itself.

Risks and Considerations

- Nutrient Deficiencies: Juice cleanses often lack essential nutrients like protein, fiber, and healthy fats, which are crucial for maintaining muscle mass, digestive health, and overall well-being.

- Blood Sugar Spikes: Juices, especially those made primarily from fruits, can cause rapid increases in blood sugar levels due to their high natural sugar content and lack of fiber.

- Unsustainable Weight Loss: Any weight loss experienced during a juice cleanse is typically temporary and primarily due to water loss and muscle depletion rather than fat loss.

- Potential Health Complications: Prolonged juice cleanses can lead to more serious health issues, including electrolyte imbalances, weakened immune function, and disrupted metabolic processes.

Healthier Alternatives to Juice Cleanses

Instead of relying on juice cleanses for detoxification, there are healthier and more sustainable ways to support the body's natural detox processes:

- Balanced Diet: Consuming a diet rich in whole foods, including fruits, vegetables, lean proteins, whole grains, and healthy fats, provides the nutrients needed for optimal detoxification.

- Regular Exercise: Physical activity increases blood circulation and promotes sweating, aiding in the elimination of toxins through the skin.

- Adequate Hydration: Drinking plenty of water supports kidney function and helps flush out waste products.

- Limiting Exposure to Toxins: Reducing the intake of processed foods, alcohol, and environmental pollutants can decrease the toxin load on the body.

While juicing can be a healthy addition to a balanced diet, relying solely on juices for detoxification is not supported by scientific evidence and can pose health risks. It's essential to maintain a comprehensive approach to health that includes a variety of nutrient-dense foods, regular physical activity, and adequate hydration. For individuals with specific health conditions like lupus, it is particularly important to consult with healthcare professionals before undertaking any form of dietary cleanse or significant change in eating habits.

In summary, juicing for detoxification may offer some benefits in terms of nutrient intake and hydration, but it is not a necessary or scientifically proven method for detoxifying the body. A more balanced and holistic approach to health and wellness is recommended for long-term benefits and overall well-being.

Juicing for weight loss

Juicing for weight loss is a trend that has been embraced by many looking to shed extra pounds quickly. It involves consuming primarily fruit and vegetable juices in place of meals to reduce calorie intake while still providing the body with essential nutrients. However, it's important to delve into the details of this approach to understand its potential benefits and drawbacks fully.

The Concept of Juicing for Weight Loss

The idea behind juicing for weight loss is simple: by replacing solid foods with juice, you consume fewer calories while still getting a high concentration of vitamins, minerals, and other beneficial compounds found in fruits and vegetables. This can lead to a calorie deficit, which is necessary for weight loss.

Potential Benefits

- Caloric Reduction: Juices generally contain fewer calories than the meals they replace, which can help create the calorie deficit needed for weight loss.

- Nutrient-Rich: Fresh juices provide a plethora of nutrients that can support overall health during a weight loss regimen.

- Hydration: Juicing increases water intake, which is beneficial for metabolic processes and can aid in weight loss.

The Reality of Juicing for Weight Loss

While the concept seems straightforward, the reality is more complex. There is no scientific evidence that juicing is more effective for weight loss than other calorie-restricted diets. Moreover, the weight loss experienced during a juice cleanse is often temporary and can be attributed to a loss of water weight and muscle mass rather than fat.

Risks and Drawbacks

- Nutrient Imbalance: Juices lack essential nutrients like protein, fiber, and healthy fats, which are crucial for a balanced diet.

- Short-term Results: Many people regain the weight they lost once they resume their regular diet.

- Blood Sugar Spikes: Fruit juices can cause rapid increases in blood sugar levels due to their high sugar content and lack of fiber.

- Potential for Nutritional Deficiencies: Extended periods of juicing can lead to deficiencies in vital nutrients, negatively affecting overall health.

A Closer Look at the Science

Research indicates that juice diets may lead to rapid weight loss in the short term, especially when they are very low in calories. However, these diets are not sustainable and may lead to side effects such as fatigue or nutritional deficiencies. Often, people who try juice fasts for weight loss regain the weight when the diet ends, which can contribute to a cycle of yo-yo dieting.

Sustainable Weight Loss Strategies

For those seeking long-term weight loss, it's essential to adopt sustainable habits rather than quick fixes like juice cleanses. These include:

- Balanced Diet: Incorporating a variety of whole foods, including lean proteins, whole grains, and healthy fats, along with fruits and vegetables.

- Regular Physical Activity: Engaging in regular exercise to increase calorie burn and build muscle mass.

- Mindful Eating: Paying attention to hunger cues and eating in response to physical rather than emotional needs.

The Role of Juicing in a Balanced Diet

Juicing can play a role in a balanced diet when used as a supplement to whole foods rather than a replacement. It can be a convenient way to increase your intake of fruits and vegetables, especially for those who struggle to consume the recommended daily amounts.

While juicing for weight loss can offer a quick fix, it is not a sustainable or balanced approach to long-term weight management. The best strategy for weight loss is a comprehensive lifestyle change that includes a balanced diet, regular physical activity, and mindful eating practices. If you choose to include juicing in your diet, do so in moderation and as part of a broader, more sustainable health plan.

For individuals with specific health conditions, such as lupus, it is crucial to consult with healthcare professionals before making significant dietary changes. They can provide personalized advice and ensure that any new approach is safe and appropriate for your specific health needs.

Anti-inflammatory juices

Anti-inflammatory juices are beverages made from fruits and vegetables known for their anti-inflammatory properties. These juices are sought after for their potential to reduce inflammation in the body, which is a natural response by the immune system to protect against injuries, infections, and other harmful stimuli. However, chronic inflammation can lead to various health issues, including arthritis, heart disease, and even some cancers. Therefore, consuming anti-inflammatory juices may be beneficial as part of a balanced diet to help manage inflammation-related conditions.

Understanding Inflammation

Inflammation is a complex biological response that involves various cell types, chemical signals, and responses. It's a protective mechanism that helps the body heal, but when it becomes chronic, it can contribute to the development of several diseases. The anti-inflammatory diet, which includes specific fruits and vegetables, aims to reduce chronic inflammation and promote overall health.

The Role of Diet in Managing Inflammation

Diet plays a crucial role in managing inflammation. Certain foods can exacerbate inflammation, while others can help reduce it. Foods high in sugar, saturated fats, and trans fats are known to promote inflammation, whereas foods rich in antioxidants and polyphenols can help reduce it. This is where anti-inflammatory juices come into play, as they can be a convenient way to consume a variety of these beneficial compounds.

Ingredients Commonly Found in Anti-Inflammatory Juices

Anti-inflammatory juices often include ingredients such as:

- Turmeric: Contains curcumin, a compound with potent anti-inflammatory properties.

- Ginger: Has gingerol, which has been shown to reduce inflammation-related pain.

- Berries: Rich in antioxidants and vitamins that can help reduce inflammation.

- Leafy Greens: High in vitamin E, which has been shown to protect the body from pro-inflammatory molecules called cytokines.

- Pineapple: Contains bromelain, an enzyme that may help reduce inflammation and aid in digestion.

Scientific Evidence Supporting Anti-Inflammatory Juices

Research has shown that certain compounds in fruits and vegetables can have anti-inflammatory effects. For example, the flavonoids in berries, the carotenoids in carrots, and the nitrates in leafy greens all have properties that can reduce inflammation. Studies have also indicated that regular consumption of these nutrients through juicing can contribute to a reduction in inflammation markers in the body.

Potential Benefits of Anti-Inflammatory Juices

Consuming anti-inflammatory juices may offer several health benefits, including:

- Reduced Risk of Chronic Diseases: By reducing inflammation, these juices may lower the risk of chronic diseases associated with inflammation.

- Improved Joint Health: They may help alleviate symptoms of inflammatory joint conditions like arthritis.

- Enhanced Recovery: Athletes may find that these juices help reduce muscle soreness and speed up recovery after intense workouts.

- Better Digestive Health: Ingredients like ginger and pineapple can aid digestion and reduce inflammation in the gut.

How to Incorporate Anti-Inflammatory Juices into Your Diet

To reap the benefits of anti-inflammatory juices, consider the following tips:

- Moderation: Juices should complement a diet rich in whole foods, not replace them.

- Variety: Rotate ingredients to get a broad spectrum of nutrients.

- Whole Foods: Whenever possible, include the whole fruit or vegetable to retain fiber.

- Consultation: Speak with a healthcare provider, especially if you have a condition like lupus, to ensure that juicing is appropriate for you.

Preparing Anti-Inflammatory Juices

When preparing anti-inflammatory juices, it's essential to use fresh, organic produce to avoid pesticides and other chemicals that can contribute to inflammation. Here are some steps to make your own anti-inflammatory juice:

1. Select Your Ingredients: Choose a combination of fruits and vegetables known for their anti-inflammatory properties.

2. Wash Thoroughly: Clean all produce to remove any dirt or contaminants.

3. Juice: Use a juicer to extract the juice from the produce. If you don't have a juicer, a blender can work, but you may need to strain the mixture to remove the pulp.

4. Serve Immediately: Drink the juice fresh to ensure you're getting the maximum amount of nutrients.

Anti-inflammatory juices can be a delicious and nutritious addition to a balanced diet aimed at reducing inflammation. While they are not a cure-all, they can provide a concentrated source of anti-inflammatory compounds that may help manage inflammation-related conditions. As with any dietary change, it's important to consult with a healthcare professional to ensure it's suitable for your individual health needs, especially if you have a condition like lupus.

In summary, anti-inflammatory juices offer a natural way to support the body's inflammation response, potentially leading to improved health outcomes. By understanding the ingredients and their benefits, as well as how to properly incorporate these juices into your diet, you can make an informed decision about whether they are right for you.

Juicing for energy and vitality

Juicing has become a popular way to consume nutrients, with many people turning to it for a boost in energy and vitality. This method of consuming fruits and vegetables can provide a concentrated dose of vitamins, minerals, and antioxidants, which are essential for maintaining high energy levels and overall health. In this detailed exploration, we'll delve into the benefits of juicing for energy and vitality, the best ingredients to use, and some tips to maximize the health advantages.

The Benefits of Juicing for Energy and Vitality

Natural Energy Boost: Juicing can offer a quick, natural boost of energy. Unlike caffeinated beverages that can lead to a crash, the natural sugars in fruits and vegetables provide a steady release of energy. This is due to the presence of complex carbohydrates, which are broken down slowly in the body, providing a sustained energy source.

High Nutrient Density: Juices are packed with a high concentration of nutrients. By removing the fiber during the juicing process, the body can absorb these nutrients more quickly. This can be especially beneficial in the morning or before a workout when you need an immediate energy boost.

Hydration: Juices are high in water content, which can help keep you hydrated. Proper hydration is crucial for maintaining energy levels as even mild dehydration can lead to fatigue.

Antioxidants: Juicing provides a rich source of antioxidants, which can protect the body from oxidative stress and inflammation, both of which can drain energy levels. Antioxidants also support the immune system, which is important for overall vitality.

Best Ingredients for Juicing

When it comes to juicing for energy and vitality, the ingredients you choose are crucial. Here are some of the best options:

Leafy Greens: Spinach, kale, and Swiss chard are excellent for juicing. They're high in iron, which is essential for the production of energy in the body. They also contain B vitamins, which play a key role in converting food into energy.

Citrus Fruits: Oranges, lemons, and limes are high in vitamin C, which is not only great for the immune system but also helps in the absorption of iron from plant sources, making them a perfect addition to green juices.

Beets: Rich in nitrates, beets can improve blood flow and increase oxygen delivery throughout the body, enhancing energy levels and stamina.

Apples: Apples are a good source of soluble fiber, which can help regulate blood sugar levels, preventing the spikes and crashes that can affect your energy.

Ginger: Known for its anti-inflammatory properties, ginger can also help boost circulation, contributing to increased energy and vitality.

Tips for Juicing

Balance Your Ingredients: While juicing primarily fruits can lead to a high intake of sugars, balancing fruits with vegetables can provide the sweetness you crave without the sugar overload. Aim for a higher ratio of vegetables to fruits in your juices.

Consume Immediately: To get the most benefits from juicing, consume your juice immediately after making it. This ensures that the nutrients do not degrade over time, which can happen even with refrigeration.

Listen to Your Body: Everyone's body is different, and certain ingredients may work better for some than others. Pay attention to how your body reacts to different juices and adjust your recipes accordingly.

Consult with a Healthcare Provider: If you have any health concerns or are taking medications, it's important to consult with a healthcare provider before starting a juicing regimen. Some ingredients can interact with medications or may not be suitable for certain health conditions.

Juicing for energy and vitality can be a beneficial addition to a balanced diet. It provides a natural, nutrient-rich way to boost energy levels and support overall health. By choosing the right ingredients and following the tips provided, you can maximize the benefits of juicing and enjoy the increased energy and vitality that comes with it.

Remember, while juicing can be a great way to supplement your diet with additional nutrients, it should not replace whole foods entirely. Whole fruits and vegetables provide fiber and other benefits that are not present in juice. Therefore, juicing should be used in conjunction with a diet rich in a variety of whole foods to ensure a balanced intake of all necessary nutrients.

In summary, juicing is a convenient and effective way to increase your intake of essential nutrients, hydrate your body, and give you a natural energy boost. With the right approach, it can be a valuable tool in your quest for a healthier, more vibrant life.

This exploration into the world of juicing for energy and vitality is just the beginning. There's a wealth of information and recipes available for those looking to dive deeper into this nutritious practice. Whether you're a seasoned juicer or just starting out, the potential benefits for your health and energy levels are well worth the effort. Happy juicing!

Chapter 4

Recipes

Green juices

Green juices are a cornerstone of healthful living, providing a concentrated source of nutrients that can be easily absorbed by the body. They are an excellent way to increase your intake of vegetables, particularly leafy greens, which are rich in vitamins, minerals, and antioxidants. Below, I will expound on the concept of green juices, their benefits, and provide a variety of recipes for you to try.

Understanding Green Juices

Green juices are made by extracting the juice from green vegetables and, often, fruits. The "green" in green juices typically comes from leafy green vegetables like spinach, kale, and chard, which are known for their health-promoting properties. These juices are an integral part of many health-conscious individuals' diets because they are low in calories but high in nutrients.

The Benefits of Green Juices

The benefits of consuming green juices are manifold. They are packed with chlorophyll, which is the pigment that gives plants their green color and is thought to have numerous health benefits, including detoxification and anti-inflammatory properties. Green juices are also a great source of enzymes that can aid in digestion and help promote gut health.

Moreover, green juices can contribute to better hydration and provide a quick energy boost without the crash associated with caffeinated beverages. They can also help in weight management efforts, as they are low in calories yet can be quite filling due to their high fiber content.

Crafting the Perfect Green Juice

When it comes to making green juices, the possibilities are endless. Here are some recipes to get you started, each with its unique blend of flavors and health benefits:

The Classic Cleanser

- Ingredients:

  - 2 cups of spinach

  - 1 cup of kale

- 1 green apple

- 1/2 a lemon, peeled

- 1 inch of ginger root

- Instructions:

1. Wash all ingredients thoroughly.

2. Core the apple and cut into wedges.

3. Juice all ingredients, starting with the leafy greens, followed by the apple, lemon, and ginger.

4. Stir the juice and serve immediately.

The Immune Booster

- Ingredients:

- 1 cup of Swiss chard

- 1/2 a cucumber

- 2 stalks of celery

- 1/2 a green bell pepper

- 1/2 a lime, peeled

- Instructions:

1. Clean all produce.

2. Juice the Swiss chard and celery, followed by the cucumber and bell pepper.

3. Finish with the lime for a zesty kick.

4. Enjoy the juice fresh for the best nutrient intake.

The Sweet Green

- Ingredients:

- 1 handful of romaine lettuce

- 1/2 a pear

- 1/2 a kiwi

- 1/2 a cup of pineapple

- A sprig of mint

- Instructions:

1. Rinse all fruits and vegetables.

2. Juice the romaine, pear, and kiwi.

3. Add the pineapple and mint last for a refreshing flavor.

4. Serve chilled for a sweet treat.

The Spicy Detox

- Ingredients:

  - 2 cups of arugula

  - 1/2 a jalapeño, seeds removed

  - 1/2 a fennel bulb

  - 1 green apple

  - 1/2 a lemon, peeled

- Instructions:

1. Thoroughly wash all ingredients.

2. Start by juicing the arugula and fennel.

3. Add the jalapeño and apple for a spicy-sweet combination.

4. Finish with lemon to balance the flavors.

5. Drink immediately to kickstart your metabolism.

The Herbal Healer

- Ingredients:

  - 1 cup of collard greens

  - 1/2 a cup of parsley

  - 1/2 a cup of cilantro

- 1 cucumber

- 1/2 a lime, peeled

- Instructions:

  1. Cleanse all herbs and vegetables.

  2. Juice the collard greens and herbs first to extract their essence.

  3. Follow with the cucumber for added hydration.

  4. Squeeze in the lime for a citrusy finish.

  5. Savor the juice for its detoxifying properties.

The Green Giant

- Ingredients:

  - 2 cups of kale

  - 1/2 a broccoli stem

  - 1 green apple

  - 1/2 a lemon, peeled

  - 1 inch of ginger root

- Instructions:

  1. Wash all produce well.

  2. Juice the kale and broccoli stem for a nutrient-rich base.

  3. Add the apple for sweetness and the lemon for tartness.

  4. Include the ginger for a warming effect.

  5. Drink this juice to feel like a green giant.

Tips for Green Juicing

- Use Fresh Ingredients: The fresher your produce, the more flavorful and nutrient-dense your juice will be.

- Balance Flavors: Combine bitter greens with sweet fruits or acidic citrus to create a well-balanced juice.

- Juice Leafy Greens First: This ensures you get the most juice out of them before adding in other ingredients.

- Drink Immediately: To benefit from the maximum amount of nutrients, consume your green juice shortly after making it.

- Experiment: Don't be afraid to try new combinations and find what you enjoy the most.

Green juices are a simple yet powerful way to boost your health. By incorporating a variety of greens, fruits, and herbs, you can create delicious juices that not only taste great but also provide numerous health benefits. Whether you're looking to detoxify, boost your immune system, or simply increase your vegetable intake, green juices are an excellent choice. So, grab your juicer and start exploring the wonderful world of green juices today!

Fruit juices

Fruit juices are a delightful and refreshing way to enjoy the essence of fruits in a liquid form. They are not only delicious but also packed with vitamins, minerals, and antioxidants that can provide numerous health benefits. In this detailed exploration, we will delve into the world of fruit juices, understand their benefits, and learn how to make a variety of fruit juice recipes.

The Joy of Fruit Juices

Fruit juices are more than just beverages; they are a celebration of nature's bounty. Each fruit brings its unique flavor profile, color, and nutritional benefits to the table. Juicing fruits allows us to consume a concentrated amount of these nutrients in an easily digestible form. Whether you're looking for a quick energy boost, a way to hydrate, or to increase your intake of essential nutrients, fruit juices are an excellent choice.

Nutritional Benefits

Fruits are nature's candy, rich in essential nutrients that our bodies need to function optimally. When juiced, these nutrients become readily available for our bodies to absorb:

- Vitamins: Such as vitamin C, which is crucial for immune function, and vitamin A, important for vision and skin health.

- Minerals: Like potassium, which helps maintain healthy blood pressure, and magnesium, which is involved in over 300 biochemical reactions in the body.

- Antioxidants: Compounds that protect our cells from damage caused by free radicals.

- Phytonutrients: Plant compounds that have various health benefits, including anti-inflammatory and anti-cancer properties.

The Art of Juicing

Juicing is a simple process, but there are a few tips to ensure you get the most out of your fruits:

- Use Fresh Produce: Always choose fresh, ripe fruits for the best flavor and nutrient content.

- Preparation: Wash all fruits thoroughly, and depending on the type of juicer you have, you may need to peel or chop the fruits.

- Juicing Method: Use a good quality juicer or blender to extract the juice. If using a blender, you may need to strain the juice afterward to remove the pulp.

- Consumption: Drink your juice as soon as possible after making it to enjoy the maximum nutritional benefits.

Delightful Fruit Juice Recipes

Now, let's explore some delightful fruit juice recipes that you can make at home:

1. Sunshine Citrus Juice

- Ingredients:

  - 2 oranges

  - 1 grapefruit

  - 1 lemon

- Instructions:

  1. Peel the citrus fruits and remove any seeds.

  2. Juice all the fruits together.

  3. Serve immediately to enjoy a vitamin C-packed drink.

2. Tropical Bliss

- Ingredients:

  - 1 cup pineapple chunks

  - 1 mango, peeled and pitted

  - 1/2 banana

- Instructions:

1. Blend all the ingredients until smooth.

2. Strain through a fine mesh sieve for a clear juice.

3. Enjoy this tropical delight chilled.

3. Berry Antioxidant Boost

- Ingredients:

  - 1 cup strawberries

  - 1/2 cup blueberries

  - 1/2 cup raspberries

- Instructions:

  1. Wash the berries thoroughly.

  2. Juice or blend the berries together.

  3. Serve this antioxidant-rich juice fresh.

4. Green Apple Ginger Zing

- Ingredients:

  - 2 green apples

  - 1-inch piece of ginger

  - Juice of 1/2 lemon

- Instructions:

  1. Core the apples and peel the ginger.

  2. Juice the apples and ginger, then add the lemon juice.

  3. Stir well and enjoy the zesty flavor.

5. Pomegranate Perfection

- Ingredients:

  - Seeds from 1 pomegranate

- 1 apple

- Juice of 1/2 lemon

- Instructions:

  1. Juice the pomegranate seeds and apple together.

  2. Stir in the lemon juice.

  3. Enjoy this heart-healthy juice.

6. Kiwi Cucumber Refresh

- Ingredients:

  - 3 kiwis, peeled

  - 1 cucumber

  - Juice of 1/2 lime

- Instructions:

  1. Juice the kiwis and cucumber.

  2. Add the lime juice for a refreshing twist.

  3. Serve this digestive-friendly juice chilled.

7. Peachy Keen

- Ingredients:

  - 2 ripe peaches, pitted

  - 1 cup orange juice

  - 1/2 teaspoon of honey (optional)

- Instructions:

  1. Blend the peaches with the orange juice until smooth.

  2. Sweeten with honey if desired.

  3. Serve this sweet and nourishing juice immediately.

8. The Classic Orange Juice

- Ingredients:

  - 4-5 large, ripe oranges

- Instructions:

  1. Roll the oranges on the countertop to loosen the juice inside.

  2. Cut the oranges in half and use a hand juicer or a citrus press to squeeze out the juice.

  3. Strain the juice to remove any pulp or seeds, if desired.

  4. Serve the juice immediately over ice for a refreshing drink.

9. Tropical Pineapple-Mango Juice

- Ingredients:

  - 1 ripe mango, peeled and pitted

  - 1 cup of fresh pineapple chunks

  - 1/2 cup of coconut water

- Instructions:

  1. Combine the mango and pineapple chunks in a blender.

  2. Add the coconut water for a tropical flavor and to aid blending.

  3. Blend until smooth.

  4. Strain through a fine mesh sieve for a smoother juice, if preferred.

  5. Enjoy this tropical juice chilled.

10. Berry Medley Juice

- Ingredients:

  - 1 cup of strawberries, hulled

  - 1/2 cup of raspberries

  - 1/2 cup of blueberries

  - 1 apple, cored and sliced

- 1 tablespoon of honey (optional)

- Instructions:

1. Wash all the berries and apple thoroughly.

2. Place all the ingredients in a blender and blend until smooth.

3. Strain the mixture to remove the seeds and pulp for a silkier texture.

4. Add honey for additional sweetness if needed.

5. Serve this antioxidant-rich juice immediately.

11. Green Apple and Kiwi Juice

- Ingredients:

  - 2 green apples

  - 3 kiwis, peeled

  - 1/2 lemon, peeled

  - 1-inch piece of ginger, peeled

- Instructions:

1. Core the apples and cut them into wedges.

2. Slice the kiwis and lemon.

3. Juice the apples, kiwis, lemon, and ginger through a juicer.

4. Stir the juice well and serve over ice for a zesty and refreshing drink.

12. Watermelon Mint Juice

- Ingredients:

  - 4 cups of seedless watermelon, cubed

  - A handful of fresh mint leaves

  - Juice of 1 lime

- Instructions:

1. Place the watermelon cubes in a blender.

2. Add the fresh mint leaves and lime juice.

3. Blend until smooth.

4. Strain the juice for a clear liquid, or leave as is for a more fiber-rich drink.

5. Serve the juice chilled for a hydrating and cooling beverage.

These recipes are just a starting point, and you can always adjust the ingredients according to your taste preferences and the fruits you have available. Remember to use fresh, ripe fruits for the best flavor and nutritional value. Enjoy your homemade fruit juices!

Fruit juices are a wonderful way to enjoy the natural sweetness and health benefits of fruits. With these recipes, you can easily make a variety of juices at home, each offering a unique taste and nutritional profile. Whether you're looking for a refreshing summer drink or a health-boosting elixir, these fruit juice recipes are sure to delight your palate and contribute to your well-being. So, grab your juicer or blender and start experimenting with the endless possibilities that fruit juices offer. Cheers to your health

Vegetable juices

Vegetable juices are a cornerstone of a healthy diet, offering a concentrated source of nutrients and a convenient way to increase your intake of vegetables. They can be an excellent addition to any wellness routine, providing a range of benefits from boosting immunity to aiding digestion. Let's delve into the world of vegetable juices, exploring their nutritional value, potential health benefits, and some popular vegetable juice recipes.

Nutritional Value of Vegetable Juices

Vegetable juices are packed with vitamins, minerals, antioxidants, and phytonutrients. The exact nutritional content varies depending on the vegetables used, but most are low in calories and high in essential nutrients. For example, dark leafy greens like kale and spinach are rich in vitamins A, C, and K, as well as iron and calcium. Root vegetables like carrots and beets are excellent sources of vitamin A, potassium, and manganese.

Health Benefits of Vegetable Juices

The health benefits of vegetable juices are numerous. They can help to:

- Boost Immune Function: Vegetables like bell peppers and spinach are high in vitamin C, which is known to support the immune system.

- Improve Digestion: The natural enzymes in fresh vegetable juices can aid in digestion and help alleviate issues like bloating and constipation.

- Support Heart Health: Ingredients such as beets and leafy greens are beneficial for heart health due to their high nitrate content, which can help to lower blood pressure.

- Enhance Skin Health: The antioxidants in vegetables can help to protect the skin from damage and improve its overall appearance.

- Aid in Detoxification: Juicing can support the body's natural detoxification processes by providing a high dose of nutrients that are easy to absorb.

Popular Vegetable Juice Recipes

Here are some popular vegetable juice recipes that are not only nutritious but also delicious:

- Classic Carrot Juice: Carrots are a juicing favorite due to their natural sweetness and high nutrient content. A simple carrot juice can be made by juicing carrots with a bit of ginger for added spice and digestive benefits.

- Beetroot Bliss: Beets are known for their vibrant color and earthy flavor. They pair well with apples, carrots, and a hint of lemon. Beets are particularly good for endurance and cognitive function due to their nitrate content.

- Green Goodness: A combination of cucumber, celery, green apple, and a handful of spinach or kale makes for a refreshing and nutrient-dense green juice. This juice is perfect for a midday energy boost.

Tips for Making Vegetable Juices

When making vegetable juices, there are a few tips to keep in mind:

- Use Fresh, Organic Produce: To get the most benefits from your juices, use fresh and organic vegetables whenever possible to avoid pesticides and other chemicals.

- Balance Flavors: While vegetables are the main ingredient, adding a small amount of fruit can help balance the flavors and add a touch of sweetness.

- Include a Variety of Vegetables: To ensure a wide range of nutrients, include a variety of different vegetables in your juices.

- Drink Immediately: Vegetable juices are best consumed immediately after juicing to maximize nutrient intake before oxidation occurs.

1. Carrot Ginger Zinger:

Ingredients:

- 5 large carrots

- 1-inch piece of ginger

Instructions:

1. Wash and peel the carrots.

2. Scrub the ginger root and remove the skin.

3. Cut the carrots and ginger into chunks that will fit your juicer.

4. Feed the carrots and ginger through the juicer.

5. Stir the juice and serve immediately for the best taste and nutrient retention.

2. Beetroot and Berry:

Ingredients:

- 2 medium beetroots

- 1 cup mixed berries (strawberries, blueberries, raspberries)

Instructions:

1. Wash the beetroots thoroughly and peel if desired.

2. Wash the berries and remove any stems.

3. Cut the beetroots into smaller pieces.

4. Juice the beetroots first, then follow with the berries.

5. Mix the juices well and enjoy!

3. Spicy Tomato:

Ingredients:

- 4 ripe tomatoes

- 2 stalks of celery

- A dash of hot sauce or a pinch of cayenne pepper

Instructions:

1. Wash the tomatoes and celery.

2. Cut the tomatoes into quarters and the celery into 3-inch pieces.

3. Juice the tomatoes and celery together.

4. Add the hot sauce or cayenne pepper to the juice and stir well.

5. Serve chilled for a refreshing kick.

4. Cucumber Mint:

Ingredients:

- 1 large cucumber

- A handful of fresh mint leaves

Instructions:

1. Wash the cucumber and mint leaves.

2. Cut the cucumber into strips that will fit your juicer.

3. Alternate feeding cucumber strips and mint leaves into the juicer.

4. Stir the juice to distribute the mint flavor.

5. Serve over ice for a cooling beverage.

5. Sweet Potato Delight:

Ingredients:

- 2 medium sweet potatoes

- A pinch of cinnamon

Instructions:

1. Wash and peel the sweet potatoes.

2. Cut the sweet potatoes into chunks.

3. Sprinkle cinnamon over the sweet potato chunks.

4. Juice the sweet potato chunks.

5. Serve warm or chilled, as preferred.

6. Kale and Apple Juice

Ingredients:

- 4 large kale leaves

- 2 green apples

- 1 cucumber

- 1/2 lemon (peeled)

- 1-inch piece of ginger (optional)

Instructions:

1. Wash all the ingredients thoroughly.

2. Remove the stems from the kale leaves.

3. Core the apples and cut them into quarters.

4. Cut the cucumber into chunks.

5. If using ginger, peel it and cut into smaller pieces.

6. Start by juicing the kale leaves, followed by the apples, cucumber, and ginger.

7. Finally, add the lemon for a citrusy touch.

8. Stir the juice well and serve immediately.

7. Celery Cleanse Juice

Ingredients:

- 6 celery stalks

- 1/2 lemon (peeled)

- 1 green apple (optional for sweetness)

Instructions:

1. Wash the celery stalks and apple thoroughly.

2. Cut the celery stalks into smaller pieces if needed to fit into your juicer.

3. Core the apple and cut into quarters if using.

4. Start by juicing the celery, followed by the apple, and finish with the lemon.

5. Mix the juice well and drink immediately for maximum freshness.

8. Pepper Punch Juice

Ingredients:

- 2 red bell peppers

- 1 carrot

- 1 apple

- 1/4 teaspoon cayenne pepper (optional)

Instructions:

1. Wash all the ingredients thoroughly.

2. Core and seed the bell peppers, then cut into pieces.

3. Peel and cut the carrot into chunks.

4. Core the apple and cut into quarters.

5. Juice the bell peppers first, followed by the carrot and apple.

6. If desired, add a pinch of cayenne pepper to the juice and mix well.

7. Serve immediately for a spicy, invigorating drink.

9. Broccoli Booster Juice

Ingredients:

- 1 large broccoli stem (approximately 1 cup)

- 3 carrots

- 1 apple

Instructions:

1. Wash the broccoli stem, carrots, and apple thoroughly.

2. Cut the broccoli stem into smaller pieces.

3. Peel and cut the carrots into chunks.

4. Core the apple and cut into quarters.

5. Juice the broccoli stem first, followed by the carrots and apple.

6. Stir the juice well to ensure all flavors are combined.

7. Drink immediately for a nutrient-packed boost.

10. Spinach Citrus Juice

Ingredients:

- 2 cups spinach leaves

- 2 oranges

- 1 grapefruit

- 1/2 lemon (peeled)

Instructions:

1. Wash the spinach leaves thoroughly.

2. Peel the oranges, grapefruit, and lemon, removing as much of the white pith as possible.

3. Break the oranges and grapefruit into segments to fit into your juicer.

4. Start by juicing the spinach leaves, followed by the oranges, grapefruit, and lemon.

5. Mix the juice well to blend the flavors.

6. Serve immediately for a refreshing, vitamin C-rich drink.

11. Zucchini Zen Juice

Ingredients:

- 2 medium zucchinis

- 1 cucumber

- 1 small handful of fresh basil leaves

- 1 apple (optional for sweetness)

Instructions:

1. Wash all the ingredients thoroughly.

2. Cut the zucchinis and cucumber into chunks.

3. Core the apple and cut into quarters if using.

4. Juice the zucchinis first, followed by the cucumber, basil leaves, and apple.

5. Stir the juice well to combine all the flavors.

6. Serve immediately for a refreshing, hydrating drink.

12. Parsley Lemonade Juice

Ingredients:

- 1 large bunch of parsley (about 1 cup packed)

- 2 lemons (peeled)

- 2 apples

Instructions:

1. Wash the parsley, lemons, and apples thoroughly.

2. Peel the lemons and remove as much of the white pith as possible.

3. Core the apples and cut into quarters.

4. Juice the parsley first, followed by the lemons and apples.

5. Mix the juice well to blend all the flavors.

6. Serve immediately for a refreshing and detoxifying drink.

13. Ginger Beet Juice

Ingredients:

- 2 medium beets

- 4 carrots

- 1-inch piece of ginger

- 1 apple (optional for sweetness)

Instructions:

1. Wash the beets, carrots, ginger, and apple thoroughly.

2. Peel the beets and ginger if desired.

3. Cut the beets, carrots, and apple into chunks.

4. Juice the beets first, followed by the carrots, ginger, and apple.

5. Stir the juice well to ensure all the flavors are combined.

6. Drink immediately for a vibrant and energizing juice.

14. Carrot Cucumber Juice

Ingredients:

- 5 large carrots

- 1 cucumber

- 1 small handful of fresh mint leaves

- 1 apple (optional for sweetness)

Instructions:

1. Wash the carrots, cucumber, mint leaves, and apple thoroughly.

2. Peel and cut the carrots into chunks.

3. Cut the cucumber into chunks.

4. Core the apple and cut into quarters if using.

5. Juice the carrots first, followed by the cucumber, mint leaves, and apple.

6. Mix the juice well to combine all the flavors.

7. Serve immediately for a refreshing and hydrating drink.

15. Tomato Celery Juice

Ingredients:

- 4 medium tomatoes

- 4 celery stalks

- 1/2 lemon (peeled)

- Black pepper to taste

Instructions:

1. Wash the tomatoes, celery, and lemon thoroughly.

2. Cut the tomatoes into quarters.

3. Cut the celery into smaller pieces if needed.

4. Juice the tomatoes first, followed by the celery and lemon.

5. Add a dash of black pepper to taste and mix well.

6. Serve immediately for a savory and refreshing drink.

16. Green Goddess Juice

Ingredients:

- 2 cups kale leaves

- 2 cups spinach leaves

- 4 celery stalks

- 1 cucumber

- 1 green apple

- 1/2 lemon (peeled)

Instructions:

1. Wash all the ingredients thoroughly.

2. Remove the stems from the kale leaves.

3. Cut the cucumber and celery into chunks.

4. Core the apple and cut into quarters.

5. Juice the kale, spinach, celery, cucumber, apple, and finally the lemon.

6. Stir the juice well to combine all the flavors.

7. Serve immediately for a nutrient-rich green juice.

17. Radish Refresher Juice

Ingredients:

- 6 radishes

- 2 apples

- 1 cucumber

- 1/2 lemon (peeled)

Instructions:

1. Wash the radishes, apples, cucumber, and lemon thoroughly.

2. Trim the ends off the radishes.

3. Cut the apples into quarters and remove the cores.

4. Cut the cucumber into chunks.

5. Juice the radishes first, followed by the apples, cucumber, and lemon.

6. Mix the juice well to ensure all the flavors are combined.

7. Serve immediately for a refreshing and slightly spicy juice.

18. Squash Squirt Juice

Ingredients:

- 1 small butternut squash

- 2 carrots

- 1 apple

- A pinch of nutmeg (optional)

Instructions:

1. Wash the squash, carrots, and apple thoroughly.

2. Peel and deseed the butternut squash, then cut into chunks.

3. Peel and cut the carrots into chunks.

4. Core the apple and cut into quarters.

5. Juice the butternut squash first, followed by the carrots and apple.

6. Stir in a pinch of nutmeg if desired.

7. Mix the juice well and serve immediately for a sweet and slightly spiced drink.

19. Jicama Juice

Ingredients:

- 1 medium jicama

- 2 limes (peeled)

- A pinch of chili powder (optional)

Instructions:

1. Wash the jicama and limes thoroughly.

2. Peel the jicama and cut into chunks.

3. Peel the limes and cut into segments.

4. Juice the jicama first, followed by the limes.

5. Stir in a pinch of chili powder if desired.

6. Mix the juice well and serve immediately for a refreshing and slightly tangy drink.

20. Pumpkin Pie Juice

Ingredients:

- 1 small pumpkin

- 2 apples

- 1/2 teaspoon pumpkin pie spice (or a mix of cinnamon, nutmeg, and cloves)

Instructions:

1. Wash the pumpkin and apples thoroughly.

2. Peel and deseed the pumpkin, then cut into chunks.

3. Core the apples and cut into quarters.

4. Juice the pumpkin first, followed by the apples.

5. Stir in the pumpkin pie spice.

6. Mix the juice well and serve immediately for a delicious, autumn-inspired drink.

21. Cabbage Cooler Juice

Ingredients:

- 1/2 small red cabbage

- 2 apples

- 1-inch piece of ginger

- 1/2 lemon (peeled)

Instructions:

1. Wash the cabbage, apples, ginger, and lemon thoroughly.

2. Cut the cabbage into chunks.

3. Core the apples and cut into quarters.

4. Peel the ginger if desired and cut into smaller pieces.

5. Juice the cabbage first, followed by the apples, ginger, and lemon.

6. Mix the juice well to combine all the flavors.

7. Serve immediately for a refreshing and vibrant drink.

22. Asparagus Alkalizer Juice

Ingredients:

- 8 asparagus spears

- 2 cucumbers

- 1 lemon (peeled)

- 1 green apple (optional for sweetness)

Instructions:

1. Wash the asparagus, cucumbers, lemon, and apple thoroughly.

2. Trim the ends off the asparagus spears.

3. Cut the cucumbers into chunks.

4. Core the apple and cut into quarters if using.

5. Juice the asparagus first, followed by the cucumbers, lemon, and apple.

6. Stir the juice well to blend all the flavors.

7. Serve immediately for an alkalizing and refreshing drink.

23. Garlic Greens Juice

Ingredients:

- 2 cups mixed leafy greens (kale, spinach, chard)

- 1 clove of garlic

- 1 cucumber

- 1 green apple (optional for sweetness)

Instructions:

1. Wash the leafy greens, garlic, cucumber, and apple thoroughly.

2. Remove the stems from the leafy greens if desired.

3. Cut the cucumber into chunks.

4. Core the apple and cut into quarters if using.

5. Juice the leafy greens first, followed by the garlic, cucumber, and apple.

6. Mix the juice well to ensure all the flavors are combined.

7. Serve immediately for a potent and health-boosting drink.

24. Turnip Tonic Juice

Ingredients:

- 2 medium turnips

- 2 apples

- 1/2 lemon (peeled)

Instructions:

1. Wash the turnips, apples, and lemon thoroughly.

2. Peel the turnips if desired and cut into chunks.

3. Core the apples and cut into quarters.

4. Juice the turnips first, followed by the apples and lemon.

5. Stir the juice well to blend all the flavors.

6. Serve immediately for a refreshing and slightly spicy drink.

25. Sweet Corn Silk Juice

Ingredients:

- 2 ears of sweet corn (kernels removed)

- 1 cup coconut water

- 1 lime (peeled)

Instructions:

1. Remove the kernels from the ears of corn.

2. Wash the lime thoroughly and peel it.

3. Juice the corn kernels first, followed by the lime.

4. Pour the coconut water into the juice and stir well to combine.

5. Serve immediately for a sweet and hydrating drink.

26. Eggplant Elixir Juice

Ingredients:

- 1 small eggplant

- 2 medium tomatoes

- 1 small handful of fresh basil leaves

- 1 cucumber

Instructions:

1. Wash the eggplant, tomatoes, basil, and cucumber thoroughly.

2. Peel the eggplant if desired and cut into chunks.

3. Cut the tomatoes into quarters.

4. Cut the cucumber into chunks.

5. Juice the eggplant first, followed by the tomatoes, basil, and cucumber.

6. Mix the juice well to blend all the flavors.

7. Serve immediately for a unique and savory juice.

27. Pea Shoot Power Juice

Ingredients:

- 1 cup pea shoots

- 2 pears

- 1 small handful of fresh mint leaves

- 1/2 lemon (peeled)

Instructions:

1. Wash the pea shoots, pears, mint leaves, and lemon thoroughly.

2. Core the pears and cut into quarters.

3. Juice the pea shoots first, followed by the pears, mint leaves, and lemon.

4. Stir the juice well to combine all the flavors.

5. Serve immediately for a fresh and energizing drink.

28. Lettuce Lush Juice

Ingredients:

- 1 head of romaine lettuce

- 2 kiwis (peeled)

- 1 lime (peeled)

Instructions:

1. Wash the romaine lettuce, kiwis, and lime thoroughly.

2. Peel the kiwis and cut into chunks.

3. Peel the lime and cut into segments.

4. Juice the romaine lettuce first, followed by the kiwis and lime.

5. Mix the juice well to blend all the flavors.

6. Serve immediately for a refreshing and hydrating juice.

29. Bok Choy Bliss Juice

Ingredients:

- 1 head of bok choy

- 1 cup pineapple chunks

- 1-inch piece of ginger

Instructions:

1. Wash the bok choy, pineapple, and ginger thoroughly.

2. Cut the bok choy into smaller pieces.

3. Peel and cut the pineapple into chunks.

4. Peel the ginger if desired and cut into smaller pieces.

5. Juice the bok choy first, followed by the pineapple and ginger.

6. Stir the juice well to combine all the flavors.

7. Serve immediately for a sweet and spicy juice.

30. Collard Cool Down Juice

Ingredients:

- 6 collard green leaves

- 1 cucumber

- 1 small handful of fresh mint leaves

- 1 green apple (optional for sweetness)

Instructions:

1. Wash the collard greens, cucumber, mint leaves, and apple thoroughly.

2. Remove the stems from the collard greens if desired.

3. Cut the cucumber into chunks.

4. Core the apple and cut into quarters if using.

5. Juice the collard greens first, followed by the cucumber, mint leaves, and apple.

6. Mix the juice well to ensure all the flavors are combined.

7. Serve immediately for a refreshing and cooling drink.

Incorporating vegetable juices into your diet can be a game-changer for your health. They provide a quick and easy way to consume a variety of nutrients that might be difficult to get from whole vegetables alone. Whether you're looking for a way to boost your immune system, improve your skin, or just increase your overall vegetable intake, vegetable juices are a versatile and delicious solution.

Remember to consult with a healthcare provider before making significant changes to your diet, especially if you have any health conditions or concerns. Happy juicing!

Smoothies

Smoothies have become a staple in the diet of health-conscious individuals and those looking for a quick, nutritious meal on the go. They are versatile, delicious, and packed with nutrients that can cater to a variety of dietary needs and preferences. Let's delve into the world of smoothies, exploring their benefits, potential downsides, and how to make them a healthy part of your daily routine.

What is a Smoothie?

At its core, a smoothie is a blended beverage typically made from a combination of fruits, vegetables, liquids (such as water, milk, or juice), and other ingredients like nuts, seeds, herbs, spices, and supplements. The result is a thick, creamy drink that is both refreshing and filling.

Nutritional Benefits of Smoothies

One of the primary advantages of smoothies is their nutritional density. By combining a variety of ingredients, smoothies can provide an array of vitamins, minerals, antioxidants, fiber, and protein. They are an excellent way to consume several servings of fruits and vegetables in one sitting, which can contribute to meeting daily nutritional requirements.

Fiber Content

Unlike juices, smoothies retain the fiber from whole fruits and vegetables. Fiber is essential for maintaining a healthy digestive system, regulating blood sugar levels, and keeping you feeling full longer. This can aid in weight management and prevent overeating.

Customization and Versatility

Smoothies are highly customizable. You can tailor them to suit your taste preferences, dietary restrictions, and nutritional needs. For instance, adding leafy greens like spinach or kale can boost the vitamin and mineral content, while incorporating a scoop of protein powder or Greek yogurt can make a smoothie more satiating and support muscle repair and growth.

Hydration

Smoothies can also contribute to your daily fluid intake. Ingredients like water-rich fruits and vegetables, along with the addition of liquids like water or coconut water, help keep you hydrated throughout the day.

Potential Risks and Considerations

While smoothies offer many health benefits, there are potential downsides to consider. Commercially prepared smoothies may contain added sugars, syrups, or ice cream, which can significantly increase the calorie and sugar content. It's essential to be mindful of the ingredients used in your smoothies, especially if you're monitoring your sugar intake or managing health conditions like diabetes.

Weight Management

For those looking to manage their weight, smoothies can be a double-edged sword. On one hand, the high fiber content and the inclusion of protein can promote satiety and help control hunger. On the other hand, it's easy to inadvertently create a high-calorie drink if you're not careful with ingredient portions, especially when adding nuts, seeds, and sweeteners.

Making Healthy Smoothies at Home

To ensure your smoothies are as healthy as possible, consider the following tips:

- Use whole fruits and vegetables to maximize fiber intake.

- Opt for water, unsweetened almond milk, or low-fat dairy milk as your liquid base to keep the sugar content in check.

- Include a protein source like Greek yogurt, silken tofu, or protein powder to make your smoothie more filling.

- Be cautious with added sweeteners; rely on the natural sweetness of fruits or use a small amount of honey or maple syrup if needed.

- Experiment with herbs and spices like ginger, turmeric, or cinnamon for added flavor and health benefits without extra calories.

Incorporating Smoothies into Your Diet

Smoothies can serve various roles in your diet, from a quick breakfast option to a post-workout recovery drink. They're also a convenient way to consume nutrients for those with a busy lifestyle or for individuals who struggle to eat enough fruits and vegetables.

Smoothies are a nutritious, convenient, and versatile option that can fit into almost any diet. They offer a way to increase your intake of fruits, vegetables, and other healthful ingredients. However, it's important to be mindful of the ingredients you use to avoid turning your healthy drink into a calorie-laden dessert. By making smoothies at home and choosing your ingredients wisely, you can enjoy all the benefits they have to offer while minimizing any potential drawbacks.

Here are some recipes;

1. Banana Oat Breakfast Smoothie

  - Ingredients:

  - 1 banana

  - 1 tablespoon porridge oats

  - 80g soft fruit (strawberries, blueberries, mango)

  - 150ml milk

  - 1 teaspoon honey

  - 1 teaspoon vanilla extract

  - Instructions:

  1. Start by peeling the banana and slicing it into chunks.

  2. In a blender, add the sliced banana, porridge oats, soft fruit (like strawberries, blueberries, or mango), milk, honey, and vanilla extract.

  3. Blend all the ingredients until smooth and creamy. If the consistency is too thick, you can add a bit more milk.

4. Taste the smoothie and adjust sweetness by adding more honey if desired.

5. Pour the smoothie into a glass and serve immediately. You can also top it with a sprinkle of oats or fresh fruit for an extra touch.

2. Classic Berry Smoothie

  - Ingredients:

    - 1 cup unsweetened dairy or non-dairy milk

    - 1 cup fresh baby greens (spinach, kale)

    - 1 frozen banana

    - 1 cup frozen berries

    - ½ cup Greek yogurt

    - 2 tablespoons nut butter (almond or peanut)

    - 2 tablespoons protein powder (optional)

    - Sweetener to taste (honey, agave syrup, etc.)

  - Instructions:

    1. Pour the milk into the blender.

    2. Add the baby greens, frozen banana, frozen berries, Greek yogurt, nut butter, protein powder (if using), and sweetener of your choice.

    3. Blend the mixture until it reaches a smooth consistency. You may need to pause and scrape down the sides of the blender to ensure everything is well combined.

    4. Taste the smoothie and add more sweetener if needed.

    5. Pour the smoothie into glasses and enjoy immediately, or store it in the refrigerator for a few hours if you prefer it chilled.

3. Tropical Green Smoothie

  - Ingredients:

    - 2 cups frozen fruit (banana, mango, pineapple)

    - 1 cup liquid (coconut water, almond milk)

    - ½ cup Greek yogurt

- ½ tablespoon ground flax seeds

- ¼ cup protein powder (optional)

- A handful of greens (spinach, kale)

- Instructions:

1. Add the frozen fruits, liquid (coconut water or almond milk), Greek yogurt, ground flax seeds, protein powder (if using), and greens to the blender.

2. Blend on high speed until all ingredients are well combined and the smoothie is creamy.

3. If the consistency is too thick, add more liquid gradually until you reach your desired thickness.

4. Taste the smoothie and adjust sweetness or tartness by adding a bit of honey or lemon juice if needed.

5. Pour the smoothie into glasses, garnish with a slice of fruit or a sprinkle of flax seeds if desired, and serve immediately.

4. Mango Raspberry Smoothie

- Ingredients:

- 1 ripe banana

- ½ cup Greek yogurt

- 1 cup spinach

- 1 cup pineapple chunks

- 1 tablespoon chia seeds

- 1 cup mango chunks

- ½ cup raspberries

- Instructions:

1. Peel the banana and cut it into chunks.

2. In a blender, combine the banana chunks, Greek yogurt, spinach, pineapple chunks, chia seeds, mango chunks, and raspberries.

3. Blend on high speed until the mixture is smooth and creamy.

4. If the smoothie is too thick, you can add a splash of water or more yogurt.

5. Taste the smoothie and adjust sweetness by adding a touch of honey or maple syrup if desired.

6. Pour the smoothie into glasses, garnish with a few extra raspberries or mango chunks, and enjoy!

5. Strawberry Banana Smoothie

  - Ingredients:

    - 1 cup strawberries

    - 1 banana

    - 1 tablespoon hemp seeds

    - 1 cup milk or non-dairy alternative

  - Instructions:

    1. Wash the strawberries and remove the stems.

    2. Peel the banana and cut it into chunks.

    3. In a blender, combine the strawberries, banana chunks, hemp seeds, and milk (or non-dairy alternative).

    4. Blend until smooth and creamy.

    5. If the smoothie is too thick, add a bit more milk and blend again until desired consistency is reached.

    6. Taste the smoothie and adjust sweetness by adding a bit of honey or agave syrup if needed.

    7. Pour into glasses, garnish with a strawberry slice if desired, and serve immediately.

6. Beet Berry Smoothie

  - Ingredients:

    - 1 small beet, cooked and chopped

    - 1 cup mixed berries

    - 1 banana

    - 1 cup orange juice

    - 1 teaspoon fresh ginger, grated

  - Instructions:

    1. Begin by cooking and chopping the beet.

    2. In a blender, combine the cooked beet, mixed berries, banana, orange juice, and grated ginger.

3. Blend until smooth and creamy.

4. If the smoothie is too thick, add more orange juice or water as needed.

5. Taste and adjust the sweetness or tartness by adding honey or lemon juice if desired.

6. Pour into glasses, garnish with a slice of orange or a sprinkle of chia seeds, and enjoy!

7. Peanut Butter Banana Smoothie

  - Ingredients:

   - 2 tablespoons peanut butter

   - 1 banana

   - 1 cup kefir or yogurt

   - 1 cup spinach

  - Instructions:

   1. Add the peanut butter, banana, kefir or yogurt, and spinach to a blender.

   2. Blend until smooth and creamy.

   3. If the smoothie is too thick, add a bit of water or more kefir/yogurt.

   4. Taste and adjust sweetness by adding honey or maple syrup if desired.

   5. Pour into glasses, garnish with a drizzle of peanut butter or a sprinkle of cinnamon, and enjoy!

8. Cherry-Almond Smoothie

  - Ingredients:

   - 1 banana

   - 1 cup cherries, pitted

   - ½ cup yogurt

   - 1 cup almond milk

  - Instructions:

   1. Peel the banana and slice it.

   2. In a blender, combine the sliced banana, pitted cherries, yogurt, and almond milk.

3. Blend until smooth and creamy.

4. Adjust the thickness by adding more almond milk if needed.

5. Taste and add honey or another sweetener if desired.

6. Pour into glasses, garnish with a cherry on top, and serve chilled.

9. Green Smoothie Bowl

- Ingredients:

  - 2 cups spinach

  - 1 banana

  - 1 cup almond milk

  - Toppings: granola, seeds, fresh fruit

- Instructions:

  1. In a blender, combine the spinach, banana, and almond milk.

  2. Blend until smooth and creamy.

  3. Pour the smoothie into a bowl.

  4. Top with your favorite toppings such as granola, chia seeds, fresh fruit slices, or nuts.

  5. Serve immediately and enjoy your nutritious green smoothie bowl!

10. Tropical Oatmeal Smoothie

- Ingredients:

  - 1 cup tropical fruits (mango, pineapple, banana)

  - ¼ cup rolled oats

  - 1 cup milk or non-dairy alternative

- Instructions:

  1. In a blender, combine the tropical fruits, rolled oats, and milk (or non-dairy alternative).

  2. Blend until smooth and creamy.

  3. If the smoothie is too thick, add more milk until you reach the desired consistency.

4. Taste and add honey or agave syrup if you prefer a sweeter smoothie.

5. Pour into glasses, garnish with a slice of mango or a sprinkle of shredded coconut, and enjoy your tropical oatmeal smoothie!

11. Blueberry Muffin Smoothie

- Ingredients:

  - 1 cup blueberries

  - 1 banana

  - ¼ cup oats

  - 1 cup milk

  - 1 teaspoon vanilla extract

- Instructions:

  1. In a blender, combine the blueberries, banana, oats, milk, and vanilla extract.

  2. Blend until smooth and creamy.

  3. Taste and adjust sweetness by adding a bit of honey or maple syrup if desired.

  4. Pour into glasses, garnish with a few blueberries or a sprinkle of cinnamon, and enjoy!

12. Pineapple Coconut Smoothie

- Ingredients:

  - 1 cup pineapple chunks

  - 1 cup coconut milk

  - 1 banana

  - 1 cup ice

- Instructions:

  1. In a blender, combine the pineapple chunks, coconut milk, banana, and ice.

  2. Blend until smooth and frothy.

  3. Taste and add honey or agave syrup if you prefer a sweeter smoothie.

4. Pour into glasses, garnish with a slice of pineapple or a sprinkle of shredded coconut, and enjoy your tropical delight!

13. Chocolate Avocado Smoothie

- Ingredients:

  - 1 avocado

  - 2 tablespoons cocoa powder

  - 1 banana

  - 1 cup milk

  - 1 tablespoon honey

- Instructions:

  1. Scoop out the flesh of the avocado and add it to a blender.

  2. Add cocoa powder, banana, milk, and honey to the blender.

  3. Blend until smooth and creamy.

  4. Taste and adjust sweetness by adding more honey if needed.

  5. Pour into glasses, garnish with a sprinkle of cocoa powder or a few chocolate shavings, and enjoy your indulgent chocolate avocado smoothie!

14. Peaches and Cream Smoothie

- Ingredients:

  - 1 cup peaches, sliced

  - ½ cup vanilla yogurt

  - 1 cup milk

  - 1 tablespoon honey

- Instructions:

  1. In a blender, combine the sliced peaches, vanilla yogurt, milk, and honey.

  2. Blend until smooth and creamy.

  3. Taste and add more honey if you prefer a sweeter smoothie.

4. Pour into glasses, garnish with a peach slice or a sprinkle of cinnamon, and enjoy your peaches and cream delight!

15. Spiced Pumpkin Smoothie

- Ingredients:

  - ½ cup pumpkin puree

  - 1 banana

  - ½ cup yogurt

  - 1 cup milk

  - 1 teaspoon pumpkin spice

- Instructions:

  1. In a blender, combine the pumpkin puree, banana, yogurt, milk, and pumpkin spice.

  2. Blend until smooth and creamy.

  3. Taste and add more pumpkin spice or a dash of cinnamon if desired.

  4. Pour into glasses, garnish with a sprinkle of pumpkin spice or a cinnamon stick, and enjoy your cozy spiced pumpkin smoothie!

Remember, the key to a healthy smoothie is balance. Focus on incorporating a variety of nutrients to create a well-rounded beverage that supports your overall health and wellness goals. Enjoy the process of experimenting with different combinations and discovering your favorite smoothie recipes that not only taste great but also nourish your body.

Chapter 5

Advanced juicing

Combining juicing with other diets

Combining juicing with other diets opens up a world of possibilities for enhancing nutrition, supporting health goals, and adding variety to your meals. Whether you follow a specific dietary plan like Paleo, Keto, Vegan, or are exploring detox diets or weight loss programs, integrating juicing can be both beneficial and enjoyable.

Paleo Diet and Juicing:

The Paleo diet focuses on whole, unprocessed foods that our ancestors would have eaten, emphasizing meats, fish, vegetables, fruits, nuts, and seeds while excluding grains, legumes, and processed foods. Juicing can complement this diet by providing concentrated nutrients from fruits and vegetables. However, it's important to avoid excessive sugar intake from high-sugar fruits in juices. Opt for lower-sugar options like green vegetables (spinach, kale, celery), cucumbers, lemon, and berries (blueberries, raspberries). You can also add healthy fats like avocado or coconut oil to your juices for a Paleo-friendly boost.

Paleo-Friendly Juice:

Ingredients:

- 1 cucumber

- 1 cup spinach

- 1 cup kale

- 1/2 lemon, peeled

- 1/2 cup blueberries

- 1 tablespoon avocado or coconut oil (optional)

- Ice cubes (optional)

Instructions:

1. Wash the cucumber, spinach, and kale thoroughly.

2. Cut the cucumber into chunks.

3. In a juicer, combine cucumber chunks, spinach, kale, peeled lemon, and blueberries.

4. If using, add avocado or coconut oil to the juicer.

5. Process the ingredients until smooth.

6. Add ice cubes if desired for a chilled drink.

7. Pour into a glass and enjoy your Paleo-friendly juice!

These recipes provide nutritious and flavorful options that align with specific diets, supporting your health goals while adding variety to your meals. Adjust ingredients based on personal preferences and dietary requirements, and enjoy the benefits of juicing as part of a balanced diet.

Keto Diet and Juicing:

The Keto diet is a low-carbohydrate, high-fat diet designed to induce ketosis, a metabolic state where the body burns fat for fuel. Juicing on Keto requires careful selection of ingredients to keep carbs low while providing essential nutrients. Focus on low-carb vegetables like leafy greens (spinach, kale, Swiss chard), celery, cucumber, and cruciferous vegetables (broccoli, cauliflower). Avoid high-sugar fruits and opt for small amounts of berries or lemon/lime for flavor. You can add healthy fats like MCT oil, avocado, or coconut cream to your juices to support ketosis and enhance satiety.

Keto-Friendly Green Juice:

Ingredients:

- 1 cup spinach

- 1 cup kale

- 1 stalk celery

- 1/2 cucumber

- 1/2 lemon, peeled

- 1 tablespoon MCT oil

- Ice cubes (optional)

Instructions:

1. Wash the spinach, kale, celery, and cucumber.

2. Cut the cucumber into smaller pieces.

3. In a juicer, combine spinach, kale, celery, cucumber, and peeled lemon.

4. Add MCT oil to the juicer.

5. Process the ingredients until well blended.

6. Add ice cubes if desired.

7. Pour into a glass and enjoy your Keto-friendly green juice!

Vegan Diet and Juicing:

A Vegan diet excludes all animal products and focuses on plant-based foods like fruits, vegetables, grains, legumes, nuts, and seeds. Juicing fits seamlessly into a Vegan lifestyle, providing a convenient way to increase intake of vitamins, minerals, and antioxidants. Create vibrant juice blends with a variety of colorful fruits and vegetables. Include leafy greens, citrus fruits, apples, carrots, beets, ginger, and turmeric for a nutrient-rich boost. You can also add plant-based proteins like hemp seeds, chia seeds, or pea protein powder to your juices for added nutrition.

Vegan Nutrient-Rich Juice:

Ingredients:

- 1 apple

- 1 carrot

- 1 small piece of ginger

- 1/2 lemon, peeled

- 1 handful spinach

- 1/2 beetroot (optional)

- 1 tablespoon hemp seeds or chia seeds (optional)

- Ice cubes (optional)

Instructions:

1. Wash the apple, carrot, ginger, lemon, spinach, and beetroot.

2. Core the apple and cut it into chunks.

3. In a juicer, combine apple chunks, carrot, ginger, peeled lemon, spinach, and beetroot (if using).

4. Add hemp seeds or chia seeds to the juicer for extra nutrition.

5. Process until smooth and well blended.

6. Add ice cubes if desired.

7. Pour into a glass and enjoy your nutrient-rich Vegan juice!

Detox Diets and Juicing:

Detox diets aim to eliminate toxins from the body, support digestion, and promote overall well-being. Juicing plays a key role in detox diets by providing a concentrated source of nutrients while giving the digestive system a break. Focus on detoxifying ingredients like leafy greens (kale, spinach), cruciferous vegetables (broccoli, cabbage), herbs (parsley, cilantro), ginger, turmeric, lemon, and beetroot. These ingredients support liver function, aid in detoxification, and boost antioxidant activity. Incorporate green juices, detoxifying smoothies, and herbal teas for a comprehensive detox plan.

Detoxifying Green Juice:

Ingredients:

- 1 cup kale

- 1 cup spinach

- 1/2 cucumber

- 1/2 lemon, peeled

- 1 handful parsley or cilantro

- 1 small piece of ginger

- 1/2 beetroot (optional)

- Ice cubes (optional)

Instructions:

1. Wash the kale, spinach, cucumber, lemon, parsley or cilantro, ginger, and beetroot.

2. Cut the cucumber into smaller pieces.

3. In a juicer, combine kale, spinach, cucumber, peeled lemon, parsley or cilantro, ginger, and beetroot (if using).

4. Process until smooth and well combined.

5. Add ice cubes if desired.

6. Pour into a glass and enjoy your detoxifying green juice!

Weight Loss Diets and Juicing:

Juicing can be a valuable tool in weight loss diets by providing nutrient-dense, low-calorie options that support satiety and overall health. However, it's essential to balance ingredients to avoid excessive sugar and calorie intake. Create weight-loss-friendly juices with a base of water-rich vegetables like cucumber, celery, and leafy greens. Add a small amount of low-sugar fruits like berries, green apples, or citrus fruits for flavor. Include ingredients that promote metabolism and digestion such as ginger, lemon, cayenne pepper, and green tea. You can also add protein-rich ingredients like chia seeds, hemp seeds, or Greek yogurt to your juices for added satiety.

Weight Loss Friendly Juice:

Ingredients:

- 1 cucumber

- 1 stalk celery

- 1 cup spinach

- 1/2 green apple

- 1/2 lemon, peeled

- 1/2 inch piece of ginger

- 1/2 teaspoon cayenne pepper (optional)

- 1 cup brewed green tea (cooled)

- 1 tablespoon chia seeds or hemp seeds (optional)

- Ice cubes (optional)

Instructions:

1. Wash the cucumber, celery, spinach, green apple, lemon, and ginger.

2. Cut the cucumber and green apple into smaller pieces.

3. In a juicer, combine cucumber, celery, spinach, green apple, peeled lemon, ginger, and cayenne pepper (if using).

4. Add cooled brewed green tea to the juicer.

5. Process until smooth and well blended.

6. Add chia seeds or hemp seeds for added nutrition.

7. Add ice cubes if desired.

8. Pour into a glass and enjoy your weight-loss-friendly juice!

Tips for Combining Juicing with Other Diets:

1. Focus on Nutrient Density: Choose a variety of colorful fruits and vegetables to ensure a wide range of vitamins, minerals, and antioxidants.

2. Mindful Sugar Intake: Be cautious with high-sugar fruits in juices, especially if you're following a low-carb or Keto diet. Opt for lower-sugar options like berries, citrus fruits, and green apples.

3. Include Healthy Fats: Incorporate sources of healthy fats like avocado, coconut oil, nuts, and seeds to support satiety and nutrient absorption.

4. Hydration: Drink plenty of water alongside juices to stay hydrated, especially if you're following a detox or weight loss plan.

5. Listen to Your Body: Pay attention to how your body responds to juicing and adjust recipes accordingly. Everyone's nutritional needs and preferences are different.

Incorporating juicing into various diets can enhance nutritional intake, support health goals, and add delicious variety to meals. Experiment with different combinations, listen to your body's feedback, and enjoy the benefits of juicing as part of a balanced diet.

Chapter 6

The Significance of Hydration and Electrolyte Balance

Hydration and electrolyte balance are critical components of maintaining optimal health and physiological function. Water is essential for survival, making up about 60% of an adult's body weight and playing a vital role in numerous bodily processes. Electrolytes, including sodium, potassium, calcium, magnesium, chloride, bicarbonate, and phosphate, are minerals that dissolve in water and carry an electric charge, essential for various bodily functions. This article explores the significance of hydration and electrolyte balance, highlighting their roles in maintaining health, the consequences of imbalance, and strategies for achieving optimal hydration and electrolyte levels.

The Role of Hydration

Water is fundamental to life and is involved in nearly every bodily function. The importance of adequate hydration cannot be overstated, as it influences physical and mental performance, temperature regulation, nutrient transport, and waste elimination. Here are some of the key roles of hydration in the body:

1. Cellular Function:

Every cell in the body requires water to function properly. Water is involved in the biochemical reactions within cells, including the production of energy. It acts as a solvent, dissolving nutrients and other substances, enabling their transport into and out of cells. Adequate hydration ensures that cells maintain their shape and structural integrity, which is crucial for proper cellular function and overall health.

2. Temperature Regulation:

The body maintains its temperature through processes such as sweating and respiration, both of which rely on water. When the body overheats, sweat glands release sweat, which evaporates from the skin surface, cooling the body. This process requires sufficient water intake to replenish the lost fluids and prevent dehydration.

3. Nutrient Transport and Absorption:

Water is essential for the digestion and absorption of nutrients. It aids in breaking down food in the digestive system and dissolves nutrients, making them accessible for absorption in the intestines. Blood, which is largely composed of water, transports these nutrients to cells throughout the body.

4. Waste Removal:

The kidneys filter waste products from the blood, excreting them in urine, which is predominantly water. Adequate hydration ensures efficient waste removal, preventing the buildup of toxins in the body. Water also helps in the elimination of waste through feces, sweat, and exhaled breath.

5. Joint and Tissue Health:

Water acts as a lubricant and cushion for joints, helping to prevent friction and wear. It is a major component of synovial fluid, which lubricates joints. Hydration also supports the health of tissues, including the skin, eyes, and mucous membranes, keeping them moist and functional.

6. Cognitive Function:

Dehydration can impair cognitive function, affecting concentration, alertness, and short-term memory. Proper hydration is essential for maintaining brain function and mental performance. Even mild dehydration can lead to headaches, mood swings, and decreased cognitive ability.

The Role of Electrolytes

Electrolytes are minerals that carry an electric charge and are vital for numerous bodily functions. They are found in bodily fluids, including blood, urine, and sweat, and are essential for maintaining fluid balance, nerve function, muscle contractions, and other physiological processes. Key electrolytes include sodium, potassium, calcium, magnesium, chloride, bicarbonate, and phosphate. Here's a closer look at their roles:

1. Fluid Balance:

Electrolytes help regulate the distribution of water within the body's compartments, including intracellular (inside cells) and extracellular (outside cells) spaces. Sodium and chloride are primarily responsible for maintaining the balance of fluids outside cells, while potassium is crucial for fluid balance inside cells. This balance is essential for maintaining blood pressure and overall fluid homeostasis.

2. Nerve Function:

Electrolytes, particularly sodium, potassium, and calcium, are crucial for the transmission of nerve impulses. These minerals generate and transmit electrical signals that facilitate communication between nerves and muscles. Sodium-potassium pumps in nerve cell membranes create electrical gradients, allowing nerve impulses to travel along nerves and across synapses.

3. Muscle Contractions:

Electrolytes play a critical role in muscle contraction and relaxation. Calcium ions trigger muscle contractions by facilitating the interaction between actin and myosin, the proteins responsible for muscle movement. Potassium helps reset the muscle cells after contraction, ensuring proper muscle function and preventing cramps and spasms.

4. Acid-Base Balance:

Electrolytes help maintain the body's acid-base balance, which is essential for normal cellular function. Bicarbonate acts as a buffer, neutralizing excess acids or bases in the blood, thus maintaining a stable pH level. This balance is crucial for metabolic processes and overall health.

5. Hydration and Electrolyte Homeostasis:

The kidneys play a vital role in regulating electrolyte levels and maintaining homeostasis. They filter electrolytes from the blood, reabsorbing what the body needs and excreting the excess through urine. Hormones, such as aldosterone and antidiuretic hormone (ADH), also regulate the balance of electrolytes and water in the body.

Consequences of Imbalance

Imbalances in hydration and electrolyte levels can have significant health consequences. Both dehydration and overhydration, as well as electrolyte imbalances, can disrupt bodily functions and lead to various health issues. Here are some potential consequences:

1. Dehydration:

Dehydration occurs when the body loses more fluids than it takes in, leading to a deficit. This can result from inadequate fluid intake, excessive sweating, diarrhea, vomiting, or certain medical conditions. Symptoms of dehydration include dry mouth, thirst, dark urine, fatigue, dizziness, and confusion. Severe dehydration can lead to kidney failure, shock, and even death.

2. Overhydration (Hyponatremia):

Overhydration, or water intoxication, occurs when there is an excessive intake of water, leading to a dilution of sodium levels in the blood (hyponatremia). This can disrupt cellular function and result in symptoms such as nausea, headache, confusion, seizures, and, in severe cases, coma and death. It is often seen in endurance athletes who consume large amounts of water without adequate sodium replacement.

3. Electrolyte Imbalance:

Electrolyte imbalances can occur due to various factors, including dehydration, overhydration, kidney disease, medications, and certain medical conditions. Common imbalances include:

- Hyponatremia: Low sodium levels, leading to symptoms such as headache, nausea, confusion, and seizures.

- Hypernatremia: High sodium levels, causing symptoms like thirst, confusion, muscle twitching, and seizures.

- Hypokalemia: Low potassium levels, resulting in muscle weakness, cramps, fatigue, and irregular heart rhythms.

- Hyperkalemia: High potassium levels, leading to muscle weakness, fatigue, and potentially life-threatening cardiac arrhythmias.

- Hypocalcemia: Low calcium levels, causing muscle spasms, tingling, and, in severe cases, convulsions.

- Hypercalcemia: High calcium levels, leading to symptoms such as nausea, vomiting, constipation, and kidney stones.

4. Impact on Physical Performance:

Both dehydration and electrolyte imbalances can significantly impair physical performance. Dehydration reduces blood volume, leading to decreased cardiac output and reduced oxygen delivery to muscles. This results in early fatigue, reduced endurance, and impaired strength. Electrolyte imbalances can cause muscle cramps, weakness, and decreased coordination, further affecting performance.

Strategies for Optimal Hydration and Electrolyte Balance

Maintaining optimal hydration and electrolyte balance involves several strategies, including adequate fluid intake, balanced nutrition, and awareness of factors that affect hydration and electrolyte levels. Here are some key strategies:

1. Adequate Fluid Intake:

The amount of water needed varies based on factors such as age, gender, activity level, climate, and overall health. A general guideline is to consume at least 8 cups (2 liters) of water per day. However, individual needs may be higher, especially for athletes or those living in hot climates. It's important to listen to your body and drink when thirsty, but also to monitor the color of your urine (light yellow indicates adequate hydration).

2. Balanced Nutrition:

A balanced diet that includes a variety of fruits, vegetables, whole grains, and lean proteins can help maintain electrolyte balance. Foods rich in electrolytes include:

- Sodium: Found in table salt, processed foods, and some vegetables.

- Potassium: Abundant in bananas, oranges, potatoes, spinach, and beans.

- Calcium: Found in dairy products, leafy greens, and fortified foods.

- Magnesium: Present in nuts, seeds, whole grains, and leafy greens.

Limiting the intake of processed foods and added salts can help prevent excessive sodium intake, which is often linked to high blood pressure and other health issues.

3. Electrolyte-Rich Beverages:

For individuals who engage in intense physical activity or exercise for extended periods, consuming electrolyte-rich beverages can help replenish lost electrolytes. Sports drinks, coconut water, and oral rehydration solutions are designed to provide a balance of electrolytes and fluids. These can be particularly useful in hot and humid environments where sweat losses are significant.

4. Monitoring Hydration Status:

Regularly monitoring hydration status can help prevent dehydration and overhydration. Simple methods include checking the color of urine (clear to light yellow is ideal) and monitoring body weight changes before and after exercise (a significant loss indicates dehydration). Paying attention to signs of thirst, fatigue, and cognitive function can also provide insights into hydration status.

5. Adjusting to Environmental Conditions:

Environmental factors such as temperature, humidity, and altitude can significantly affect hydration needs. In hot and humid conditions, the body loses more water through sweat, increasing the need for fluid intake. At high altitudes, the body also loses more water through respiration. Being aware of these conditions and adjusting fluid intake accordingly is essential for maintaining hydration and electrolyte balance.

6. Recognizing and Responding to Signs of Imbalance:

Being attuned to the body's signals of dehydration or electrolyte imbalance can prevent serious health issues. Symptoms such as dry mouth, excessive thirst, dark urine, dizziness, and fatigue indicate dehydration and should be addressed promptly by increasing fluid intake. Similarly, muscle cramps, irregular heartbeats, and cognitive disturbances can signal electrolyte imbalances, necessitating dietary adjustments or electrolyte supplements.

7. Hydration During Exercise:

During physical activity, especially high-intensity or endurance exercise, the body loses significant amounts of water and electrolytes through sweat. It is crucial to hydrate before, during, and after exercise to maintain performance and prevent dehydration. Sports drinks containing electrolytes can be beneficial during prolonged exercise sessions to replace lost electrolytes and provide quick energy.

8. Special Considerations for Athletes:

Athletes have unique hydration and electrolyte needs due to the intensity and duration of their physical activities. They should:

- Pre-Hydrate: Drink plenty of fluids before exercise to start well-hydrated.

- Hydrate During Exercise: Consume fluids at regular intervals, aiming for about 7-10 ounces every 10-20 minutes.

- Post-Exercise Rehydration: Replace fluids lost during exercise by drinking 16-24 ounces of fluid for every pound of body weight lost.

9. Hydration in Illness:

Certain illnesses and medical conditions, such as fever, diarrhea, and vomiting, can lead to increased fluid and electrolyte losses. During illness, it is vital to drink plenty of fluids and consider oral rehydration solutions that contain electrolytes to prevent dehydration and restore balance.

10. Hydration for Specific Populations:

- Children: Children are more susceptible to dehydration due to their higher surface area-to-body weight ratio. Encouraging regular fluid intake, especially during play and physical activities, is essential.

- Elderly: Older adults may have a reduced sense of thirst and are at higher risk of dehydration. Ensuring they have easy access to fluids and encouraging regular drinking habits is important.

- Pregnant and Breastfeeding Women: These women have increased fluid needs to support fetal development and milk production. Adequate hydration is crucial for both maternal and fetal health.

The Science Behind Hydration and Electrolyte Balance

Understanding the physiological mechanisms that regulate hydration and electrolyte balance provides deeper insights into their significance. Here are some key scientific concepts:

1. Osmoregulation:

Osmoregulation is the process by which the body maintains the balance of water and electrolytes. It involves the kidneys, which filter blood, reabsorb needed substances, and excrete waste in the form of urine. Hormones such as antidiuretic hormone (ADH) play a crucial role in this process by regulating water reabsorption in the kidneys, thereby controlling urine concentration.

2. Sodium-Potassium Pump:

The sodium-potassium pump is a cellular mechanism that uses energy to transport sodium ions out of cells and potassium ions into cells. This pump is essential for maintaining the electrical gradient across cell membranes, which is necessary for nerve impulse transmission and muscle contractions.

3. Renin-Angiotensin-Aldosterone System (RAAS):

The RAAS is a hormone system that regulates blood pressure and fluid balance. When blood volume or sodium levels are low, the kidneys release renin, which triggers a cascade of reactions leading to the production of aldosterone. Aldosterone signals the kidneys to retain sodium and water, increasing blood volume and restoring balance.

4. Fluid Compartments:

The body's water is distributed across different compartments: intracellular fluid (inside cells) and extracellular fluid (outside cells). The extracellular fluid is further divided into interstitial fluid (between cells) and plasma (the liquid part of blood). Electrolytes play a crucial role in maintaining the osmotic balance between these compartments, ensuring proper fluid distribution and cellular function.

Hydration and Electrolyte Balance in Clinical Settings

In clinical settings, maintaining hydration and electrolyte balance is critical for patient care. Healthcare providers use various strategies to manage and monitor these parameters:

1. Intravenous (IV) Fluids:

In cases of severe dehydration or electrolyte imbalance, IV fluids are administered to quickly restore balance. IV solutions can be isotonic, hypotonic, or hypertonic, depending on the patient's needs:

- Isotonic Solutions: Such as normal saline (0.9% sodium chloride), maintain fluid balance without altering cell volume.

- Hypotonic Solutions: Such as half-normal saline (0.45% sodium chloride), help hydrate cells by drawing water into them.

- Hypertonic Solutions: Such as 3% saline, draw water out of cells and are used in specific conditions like hyponatremia.

2. Oral Rehydration Therapy (ORT):

ORT is a simple and effective treatment for dehydration, especially in cases of diarrhea. ORT solutions contain a precise balance of salts and sugars, which enhance water absorption in the intestines. This therapy is widely used in both clinical and community settings, particularly in low-resource areas.

3. Monitoring Electrolyte Levels:

Regular monitoring of electrolyte levels through blood tests is crucial for patients with conditions affecting hydration and electrolyte balance, such as kidney disease, heart failure, and endocrine disorders. These tests help guide treatment decisions and prevent complications.

4. Management of Chronic Conditions:

Patients with chronic conditions such as diabetes, hypertension, and renal disease often require careful management of hydration and electrolyte levels. Medications, dietary modifications, and regular monitoring are essential to prevent imbalances and associated complications.

The Importance of Education and Awareness

Educating the public about the importance of hydration and electrolyte balance is vital for promoting health and preventing disease. Awareness campaigns, nutritional guidelines, and public health initiatives can help individuals make informed choices about their hydration and electrolyte needs. Key educational messages include:

1. The Importance of Drinking Water:

Highlighting the benefits of regular water intake and encouraging the habit of carrying a water bottle can promote better hydration practices.

2. Recognizing Signs of Dehydration:

Educating individuals about the early signs of dehydration, such as dry mouth, fatigue, and dark urine, can help them take timely action to rehydrate.

3. Balancing Electrolytes:

Providing information about foods rich in electrolytes and the importance of a balanced diet can help individuals maintain electrolyte balance.

4. Hydration for Athletes and Active Individuals:

Tailored advice for athletes on how to stay hydrated and replenish electrolytes during and after exercise can enhance performance and prevent imbalances.

5. Special Populations:

Targeted education for vulnerable groups, such as children, the elderly, and pregnant women, can ensure they receive adequate hydration and electrolyte support.

Hydration and electrolyte balance are fundamental to health and well-being. Water and electrolytes play critical roles in maintaining cellular function, temperature regulation, nutrient transport, waste elimination, nerve function, muscle contractions, and acid-base balance. Imbalances can lead to serious health consequences, affecting physical performance, cognitive function, and overall health. By understanding the importance of hydration and electrolytes, recognizing the signs of imbalance, and adopting strategies for maintaining balance, individuals can support their health and prevent complications. Education and awareness are key to promoting healthy hydration and electrolyte practices, ensuring that everyone can enjoy the benefits of optimal hydration and electrolyte balance.

Chapter 7

Antioxidant-Rich Juices for Kidney Health

Maintaining kidney health is critical to overall wellness, as the kidneys play a crucial role in filtering waste, balancing fluids, and regulating blood pressure. Oxidative stress and inflammation are significant contributors to kidney damage and chronic kidney disease (CKD). Antioxidants, which neutralize harmful free radicals, can help protect the kidneys and support their function. Incorporating antioxidant-rich juices into the diet is a delicious and effective way to boost kidney health. This article explores the benefits of such juices and provides recipes for making them at home.

The Role of Antioxidants in Kidney Health

Oxidative stress occurs when there is an imbalance between free radicals and antioxidants in the body, leading to cellular damage. The kidneys, due to their high metabolic activity and role in detoxification, are particularly vulnerable to oxidative stress. Chronic oxidative stress can lead to inflammation, fibrosis, and progressive kidney damage.

Antioxidants can help mitigate these harmful effects by neutralizing free radicals and reducing inflammation. This is particularly important for individuals with conditions like hypertension and diabetes, which are major risk factors for kidney disease. By incorporating antioxidant-rich foods and beverages into their diets, people can support their kidney health and reduce the risk of developing kidney-related conditions.

Antioxidant-Rich Juices for Kidney Health

Here are some of the best antioxidant-rich juices for kidney health, along with recipes for making them at home:

1. Cranberry Juice

Benefits:

Cranberries are rich in antioxidants, particularly proanthocyanidins, which prevent bacteria from adhering to the urinary tract walls. This can reduce the risk of urinary tract infections (UTIs), which, if left untreated, can ascend to the kidneys and cause serious complications. Cranberry juice also has anti-inflammatory properties that help reduce oxidative stress in the kidneys.

Recipe:

Ingredients:

- 2 cups fresh or frozen cranberries

- 4 cups water

- 1-2 tablespoons honey or a sweetener of choice (optional)

- 1 lemon, juiced (optional)

Instructions:

1. Rinse the cranberries under cold water.

2. In a large pot, combine the cranberries and water. Bring to a boil.

3. Reduce heat and let it simmer for about 15 minutes or until the cranberries have burst.

4. Remove from heat and let it cool slightly.

5. Strain the mixture through a fine-mesh sieve or cheesecloth into a large bowl, pressing down on the solids to extract as much juice as possible.

6. If desired, sweeten with honey or a sweetener of choice and add lemon juice.

7. Chill in the refrigerator before serving.

2. Pomegranate Juice

Benefits:

Pomegranates are rich in antioxidants, including polyphenols, tannins, and anthocyanins. These compounds have been shown to reduce oxidative stress and inflammation, both of which are critical factors in the development of kidney disease. Pomegranate juice can also help lower blood pressure, a major risk factor for kidney damage.

Recipe:

Ingredients:

- 2 large pomegranates

Instructions:

1. Cut the pomegranates in half and submerge them in a bowl of water.

2. Gently break apart the pomegranate halves and separate the seeds from the pith. The seeds will sink to the bottom while the pith floats.

3. Drain the seeds and place them in a blender.

4. Blend on high until the seeds are broken down.

5. Strain the mixture through a fine-mesh sieve or cheesecloth into a bowl, pressing down to extract the juice.

6. Chill before serving.

3. Blueberry Juice

Benefits:

Blueberries are known for their high antioxidant content, particularly anthocyanins, which give them their deep blue color. Blueberry juice can help reduce inflammation and oxidative stress, both of which are important for maintaining kidney health. Additionally, blueberry juice may help regulate blood sugar levels and improve insulin sensitivity, which is crucial for individuals with diabetes—a major risk factor for kidney disease.

Recipe:

Ingredients:

- 2 cups fresh or frozen blueberries

- 1 cup water

- 1-2 tablespoons honey or a sweetener of choice (optional)

Instructions:

1. Rinse the blueberries under cold water.

2. Combine the blueberries and water in a blender.

3. Blend until smooth.

4. Strain the mixture through a fine-mesh sieve or cheesecloth into a bowl, pressing down to extract the juice.

5. If desired, sweeten with honey or a sweetener of choice.

6. Chill before serving.

4. Beet Juice

Benefits:

Beet juice is rich in betalains and nitrates, both of which have significant antioxidant properties. Betalains are pigments that give beets their vibrant red color and have been shown to reduce inflammation and oxidative stress. Nitrates in beet juice are converted to nitric oxide in the body, which helps relax and dilate blood vessels, improving blood flow and reducing blood pressure—an important factor for kidney health.

Recipe:

Ingredients:

- 2 medium beets, peeled and chopped

- 1 apple, cored and chopped (optional, for sweetness)

- 1-inch piece of ginger (optional, for flavor)

- 1 cup water

Instructions:

1. Combine the beets, apple, ginger, and water in a blender.

2. Blend until smooth.

3. Strain the mixture through a fine-mesh sieve or cheesecloth into a bowl, pressing down to extract the juice.

4. Chill before serving.

5. Carrot Juice

Benefits:

Carrot juice is an excellent source of beta-carotene, a potent antioxidant that the body converts to vitamin A. Vitamin A plays a vital role in maintaining the integrity of the kidney's filtering units and reducing inflammation. Carrots also contain other antioxidants, such as lutein and zeaxanthin, which further support kidney health by reducing oxidative stress.

Recipe:

Ingredients:

- 4 large carrots, peeled and chopped

- 1 apple, cored and chopped (optional, for sweetness)

- 1-inch piece of ginger (optional, for flavor)

- 1 cup water

Instructions:

1. Combine the carrots, apple, ginger, and water in a blender.

2. Blend until smooth.

3. Strain the mixture through a fine-mesh sieve or cheesecloth into a bowl, pressing down to extract the juice.

4. Chill before serving.

6. Watermelon Juice

Benefits:

Watermelon juice is packed with antioxidants like lycopene and vitamin C. Lycopene, in particular, has been shown to reduce oxidative stress and inflammation, which can protect the kidneys from damage. Watermelon also has a high water content, which helps maintain hydration and supports the kidneys in their role of filtering waste and maintaining fluid balance.

Recipe:

Ingredients:

- 4 cups watermelon, cubed and seeds removed

- Juice of 1 lime (optional, for flavor)

Instructions:

1. Combine the watermelon and lime juice in a blender.

2. Blend until smooth.

3. Strain the mixture through a fine-mesh sieve or cheesecloth into a bowl, pressing down to extract the juice.

4. Chill before serving.

7. Acai Berry Juice

Benefits:

Acai berries are known for their exceptionally high antioxidant content, particularly anthocyanins and flavonoids. Acai berry juice can help reduce oxidative stress and inflammation, thereby supporting kidney health. In addition to their antioxidant properties, acai berries have been shown to improve lipid profiles and reduce cholesterol levels, which can benefit cardiovascular health and, by extension, kidney health.

Recipe:

Ingredients:

- 2 packets of frozen acai puree (available at health food stores)

- 1 banana

- 1 cup mixed berries (e.g., blueberries, strawberries, raspberries)

- 1 cup water or coconut water

Instructions:

1. Combine the acai puree, banana, mixed berries, and water in a blender.

2. Blend until smooth.

3. Strain the mixture through a fine-mesh sieve or cheesecloth into a bowl, pressing down to extract the juice if a thinner consistency is desired.

4. Chill before serving.

Mechanisms of Action

The beneficial effects of antioxidant-rich juices on kidney health can be attributed to several mechanisms:

1. Reduction of Oxidative Stress: Antioxidants neutralize free radicals, reducing oxidative stress and preventing damage to kidney cells and tissues.

2. Anti-Inflammatory Effects: Many antioxidants possess anti-inflammatory properties, helping to reduce inflammation in the kidneys and protect against chronic kidney disease.

3. Improved Blood Flow: Some antioxidants, such as those found in beet juice, improve blood flow and reduce blood pressure, which is beneficial for kidney health.

4. Protection Against Infections: Certain juices, like cranberry juice, prevent bacterial adherence in the urinary tract, reducing the risk of infections that can affect the kidneys.

5. Regulation of Blood Sugar and Lipid Levels: Antioxidants can help regulate blood sugar and lipid levels, reducing the risk of diabetes and cardiovascular disease, which are major risk factors for kidney disease.

Potential Benefits for Specific Kidney Conditions

Chronic Kidney Disease (CKD)

CKD is characterized by the gradual loss of kidney function over time. Oxidative stress and inflammation are key contributors to the progression of CKD. Antioxidant-rich juices can help mitigate these factors, potentially slowing the progression of the disease.

For instance, studies have shown that pomegranate juice can improve renal function and reduce oxidative stress markers in patients with CKD. Similarly, cranberry juice can help prevent UTIs, which are a common complication in CKD patients.

Kidney Stones

Certain juices can also help prevent the formation of kidney stones. For example, lemon juice is rich in citric acid, which can help dissolve calcium oxalate stones and prevent their formation. While not primarily an antioxidant, the addition of lemon juice to antioxidant-rich beverages can provide additional benefits for kidney stone prevention.

Acute Kidney Injury (AKI)

Acute kidney injury (AKI) is a sudden decline in kidney function, often caused by factors like dehydration, infection, or medication toxicity. Antioxidant-rich juices can support recovery from AKI by reducing oxidative stress and promoting healing.

Beet juice, with its high nitrate content, can improve blood flow to the kidneys and support recovery from AKI. Similarly, blueberry juice can provide antioxidants that help repair damaged kidney tissues.

Additional Recipes and Variations

Mixed Berry Juice

Benefits:

Mixed berry juice combines the antioxidant properties of several berries, including blueberries, strawberries, and raspberries. This combination provides a powerful blend of vitamins, minerals, and antioxidants that support kidney health.

Recipe:

Ingredients:

- 1 cup blueberries

- 1 cup strawberries, hulled

- 1 cup raspberries

- 1 cup water

- 1 tablespoon honey or a sweetener of choice (optional)

Instructions:

1. Rinse the berries under cold water.

2. Combine the berries and water in a blender.

3. Blend until smooth.

4. Strain the mixture through a fine-mesh sieve or cheesecloth into a bowl, pressing down to extract the juice.

5. If desired, sweeten with honey or a sweetener of choice.

6. Chill before serving.

Green Juice with Antioxidants

Benefits:

Green juice made from leafy greens like spinach or kale can provide a substantial amount of antioxidants, including vitamins C and E, as well as other beneficial phytonutrients. This juice is also rich in minerals like magnesium and potassium, which are important for kidney health.

Recipe:

Ingredients:

- 1 cup spinach or kale, packed

- 1 cucumber, chopped

- 1 green apple, cored and chopped

- 1 lemon, juiced

- 1-inch piece of ginger

- 1 cup water

Instructions:

1. Rinse the spinach or kale thoroughly.

2. Combine all ingredients in a blender.

3. Blend until smooth.

4. Strain the mixture through a fine-mesh sieve or cheesecloth into a bowl, pressing down to extract the juice.

5. Chill before serving.

 Turmeric and Ginger Juice

Benefits:

Turmeric and ginger are both powerful anti-inflammatory and antioxidant agents. This juice can help reduce inflammation and oxidative stress in the kidneys, promoting overall kidney health.

Recipe:

Ingredients:

- 1-inch piece of fresh turmeric root, peeled

- 1-inch piece of fresh ginger root, peeled

- 1 carrot, peeled and chopped

- 1 orange, peeled and segmented

- 1 cup water

Instructions:

1. Combine all ingredients in a blender.

2. Blend until smooth.

3. Strain the mixture through a fine-mesh sieve or cheesecloth into a bowl, pressing down to extract the juice.

4. Chill before serving.

Considerations and Precautions

While antioxidant-rich juices offer numerous benefits for kidney health, it is important to consider a few precautions:

1. Potassium Content: Many antioxidant-rich juices, such as beet and carrot juice, are high in potassium. Individuals with advanced kidney disease or those on potassium-restricted diets should consume these juices in moderation and under medical supervision.

2. Sugar Content: Commercially available juices often contain added sugars, which can negate some of their health benefits. Opt for fresh, homemade juices or those without added sugars to maximize their positive effects.

3. Interactions with Medications: Some juices, such as grapefruit juice, can interact with medications commonly prescribed for kidney disease and other conditions. Always consult with a healthcare provider before adding new juices to your diet.

4. Oxalate Content: Certain juices, such as those from berries, can be high in oxalates, which may contribute to the formation of kidney stones in susceptible individuals. Moderation is key, and it is important to balance the intake of high-oxalate foods with those that have low oxalate levels.

Antioxidant-rich juices offer a delicious and nutritious way to support kidney health. By reducing oxidative stress, inflammation, and improving overall kidney function, these juices can play a significant role in maintaining renal health and preventing disease. Incorporating a variety of antioxidant-rich juices, such as cranberry, pomegranate, blueberry, beet, carrot, watermelon, and acai berry juice, can provide a diverse array of beneficial compounds that support kidney health.

With the provided recipes, you can easily make these health-boosting juices at home. Each recipe is designed to maximize the intake of antioxidants while being mindful of flavor and nutritional balance. As with any dietary change, it is important to consult with a healthcare professional, especially for individuals with pre-existing kidney conditions or those on specific medications. With careful consideration and moderation, antioxidant-rich juices can be a valuable addition to a kidney-friendly diet, promoting long-term renal health and overall well-being.

Chapter 8

Managing Blood Pressure and Blood Sugar Levels Through Juices

Maintaining optimal blood pressure and blood sugar levels is essential for overall health and preventing chronic diseases like hypertension, diabetes, and cardiovascular diseases. Juices made from fruits, vegetables, and other natural ingredients can play a significant role in this endeavor. This comprehensive guide explores how juices can help manage blood pressure and blood sugar levels, provides detailed recipes for making these juices at home, and explains the science behind their health benefits.

The Importance of Blood Pressure and Blood Sugar Management

Blood Pressure Management: High blood pressure, or hypertension, can lead to severe health problems, including heart disease, stroke, and kidney failure. Managing blood pressure involves maintaining a healthy diet, regular physical activity, and sometimes medication. Dietary changes, including the consumption of certain juices, can be particularly effective.

Blood Sugar Management: High blood sugar levels, or hyperglycemia, can cause serious complications, especially for individuals with diabetes. Managing blood sugar involves a balanced diet, regular exercise, and sometimes medication. Juices made from low-glycemic fruits and vegetables can help stabilize blood sugar levels.

How Juices Can Help

Juices made from specific fruits and vegetables contain vital nutrients, antioxidants, and phytochemicals that can help regulate blood pressure and blood sugar levels. These juices can:

1. Provide Essential Nutrients: Vitamins, minerals, and fiber support metabolic functions and overall health.

2. Boost Antioxidant Levels: Antioxidants combat oxidative stress and inflammation, which are linked to both high blood pressure and high blood sugar.

3. Improve Insulin Sensitivity: Certain compounds in fruits and vegetables can enhance insulin sensitivity, helping to lower blood sugar levels.

4. Support Vascular Health: Potassium and nitrates found in some vegetables help relax blood vessels, improving blood flow and reducing blood pressure.

Juice Recipes for Managing Blood Pressure

1. Spinach and Pineapple Juice

Benefits: Spinach is rich in potassium and nitrates, which help lower blood pressure. Pineapple contains bromelain, an enzyme with anti-inflammatory properties that can support cardiovascular health.

Recipe:

Ingredients:

- 2 cups fresh spinach leaves

- 1 cup fresh pineapple chunks

- 1 cucumber, peeled and chopped

- 1/2 lemon, juiced

- 1/2 cup water

Instructions:

1. Wash the spinach leaves thoroughly.

2. Combine all ingredients in a blender.

3. Blend until smooth.

4. Strain the mixture through a fine-mesh sieve or cheesecloth into a bowl.

5. Chill before serving.

2. Watermelon and Mint Juice

Benefits: Watermelon is rich in lycopene, an antioxidant that helps reduce blood pressure. It also contains citrulline, which improves blood flow. Mint adds a refreshing flavor and has anti-inflammatory properties.

Recipe:

Ingredients:

- 2 cups watermelon chunks (seeds removed)

- 1/4 cup fresh mint leaves

- 1/2 cucumber, peeled and chopped

- 1/2 lime, juiced

Instructions:

1. Combine the watermelon, mint, cucumber, and lime juice in a blender.

2. Blend until smooth.

3. Strain the mixture through a fine-mesh sieve or cheesecloth into a bowl.

4. Chill before serving.

3. Kiwi and Green Apple Juice

Benefits: Kiwi is high in potassium and vitamin C, which help lower blood pressure. Green apples provide fiber and antioxidants, supporting overall heart health.

Recipe:

Ingredients:

- 3 kiwis, peeled and chopped

- 2 green apples, cored and chopped

- 1 celery stalk, chopped

- 1/2 lemon, juiced

Instructions:

1. Combine the kiwis, green apples, celery, and lemon juice in a blender.

2. Blend until smooth.

3. Strain the mixture through a fine-mesh sieve or cheesecloth into a bowl.

4. Chill before serving.

4. Tomato and Basil Juice

Benefits: Tomatoes are rich in potassium and lycopene, which help lower blood pressure. Basil adds a unique flavor and has anti-inflammatory properties.

Recipe:

Ingredients:

- 4 ripe tomatoes, chopped

- 1/4 cup fresh basil leaves

- 1 cucumber, peeled and chopped

- 1/2 lime, juiced

Instructions:

1. Combine the tomatoes, basil, cucumber, and lime juice in a blender.

2. Blend until smooth.

3. Strain the mixture through a fine-mesh sieve or cheesecloth into a bowl.

4. Chill before serving.

5. Grapefruit and Carrot Juice

Benefits: Grapefruit contains flavonoids that help improve blood vessel function and reduce blood pressure. Carrots are rich in potassium and beta-carotene, which support heart health.

Recipe:

Ingredients:

- 1 large grapefruit, peeled and segmented

- 3 medium carrots, peeled and chopped

- 1/2 inch piece of fresh ginger

- 1/2 cup water

Instructions:

1. Combine the grapefruit, carrots, ginger, and water in a blender.

2. Blend until smooth.

3. Strain the mixture through a fine-mesh sieve or cheesecloth into a bowl.

4. Chill before serving.

Juice Recipes for Managing Blood Sugar

1. Cucumber and Lemon Juice

Benefits: Cucumbers are low in calories and carbohydrates but high in water and fiber, which helps regulate blood sugar levels. Lemon adds flavor and vitamin C, which has antioxidant properties.

Recipe:

Ingredients:

- 2 cucumbers, peeled and chopped

- 1 lemon, juiced

- 1/2 cup water

- 1 teaspoon chia seeds (optional, for added fiber)

Instructions:

1. Combine the cucumbers, lemon juice, and water in a blender.

2. Blend until smooth.

3. Strain the mixture through a fine-mesh sieve or cheesecloth into a bowl.

4. Stir in chia seeds if desired.

5. Chill before serving.

2. Bitter Gourd and Green Apple Juice

Benefits: Bitter gourd contains compounds that mimic insulin, helping to lower blood sugar levels. Green apples provide natural sweetness and fiber, aiding in blood sugar regulation.

Recipe:

Ingredients:

- 1 medium bitter gourd (karela), seeds removed and chopped

- 2 green apples, cored and chopped

- 1 cucumber, peeled and chopped

Instructions:

1. Combine the bitter gourd, green apples, and cucumber in a blender.

2. Blend until smooth.

3. Strain the mixture through a fine-mesh sieve or cheesecloth into a bowl.

4. Chill before serving.

3. Blueberry and Spinach Juice

Benefits: Blueberries are low in sugar and high in antioxidants, which can help regulate blood sugar levels. Spinach provides fiber and essential nutrients that support metabolic health.

Recipe:

Ingredients:

- 1 cup blueberries

- 2 cups fresh spinach leaves

- 1 cucumber, peeled and chopped

- 1/2 lemon, juiced

Instructions:

1. Wash the spinach leaves thoroughly.

2. Combine all ingredients in a blender.

3. Blend until smooth.

4. Strain the mixture through a fine-mesh sieve or cheesecloth into a bowl.

5. Chill before serving.

4. Cinnamon-Spiced Carrot and Orange Juice

Benefits: Carrots have a low glycemic index, and their fiber helps stabilize blood sugar levels. Oranges provide vitamin C and antioxidants. Cinnamon can help improve insulin sensitivity.

Recipe:

Ingredients:

- 3 medium carrots, peeled and chopped

- 2 oranges, peeled and segmented

- 1/2 teaspoon ground cinnamon

- 1/2 cup water

Instructions:

1. Combine the carrots, oranges, cinnamon, and water in a blender.

2. Blend until smooth.

3. Strain the mixture through a fine-mesh sieve or cheesecloth into a bowl.

4. Chill before serving.

5. Avocado and Cucumber Juice

Benefits: Avocado provides healthy fats and fiber, which help stabilize blood sugar levels. Cucumbers add hydration and additional fiber, supporting overall metabolic health.

Recipe:

Ingredients:

- 1 ripe avocado, peeled and pitted

- 2 cucumbers, peeled and chopped

- 1/2 lime, juiced

- 1/2 cup water

Instructions:

1. Combine the avocado, cucumbers, lime juice, and water in a blender.

2. Blend until smooth.

3. Strain the mixture through a fine-mesh sieve or cheesecloth into a bowl.

4. Chill before serving.

Combining Juices for Dual Benefits

Juices can be tailored to provide benefits for both blood pressure and blood sugar management by combining ingredients that target both concerns.

1. Spinach, Apple, and Beet Juice

Benefits: Spinach and beets help lower blood pressure, while apples provide fiber and natural sweetness, aiding in blood sugar regulation.

Recipe:

Ingredients:

- 2 cups fresh spinach leaves

- 1 medium beet, peeled and chopped

- 2 green apples, cored and chopped

- 1/2 lemon, juiced

Instructions:

1. Wash the spinach leaves thoroughly.

2. Combine the spinach, beet, apples, and lemon juice in a blender.

3. Blend until smooth.

4. Strain the mixture through a fine-mesh sieve or cheesecloth into a bowl.

5. Chill before serving.

2. Carrot, Celery, and Ginger Juice

Benefits: Carrots and celery help manage blood pressure due to their potassium content, while ginger adds anti-inflammatory properties and can help stabilize blood sugar levels.

Recipe:

Ingredients:

- 3 medium carrots, peeled and chopped

- 2 celery stalks, chopped

- 1-inch piece of fresh ginger, peeled and chopped

- 1/2 lemon, juiced

- 1/2 cup water

Instructions:

1. Combine the carrots, celery, ginger, lemon juice, and water in a blender.

2. Blend until smooth.

3. Strain the mixture through a fine-mesh sieve or cheesecloth into a bowl.

4. Chill before serving.

3. Tomato, Cucumber, and Spinach Juice

Benefits: Tomatoes and cucumbers help manage blood pressure due to their high potassium content. Spinach adds fiber and essential nutrients, supporting both blood pressure and blood sugar regulation.

Recipe:

Ingredients:

- 3 ripe tomatoes, chopped

- 2 cucumbers, peeled and chopped

- 2 cups fresh spinach leaves

- 1/2 lime, juiced

Instructions:

1. Wash the spinach leaves thoroughly.

2. Combine the tomatoes, cucumbers, spinach, and lime juice in a blender.

3. Blend until smooth.

4. Strain the mixture through a fine-mesh sieve or cheesecloth into a bowl.

5. Chill before serving.

4. Pomegranate, Blueberry, and Kale Juice

Benefits: Pomegranates and blueberries are rich in antioxidants that help reduce blood pressure and stabilize blood sugar levels. Kale provides fiber and essential nutrients that support metabolic health.

Recipe:

Ingredients:

- 1 cup pomegranate seeds

- 1 cup blueberries

- 2 cups fresh kale leaves

- 1/2 lemon, juiced

Instructions:

1. Wash the kale leaves thoroughly.

2. Combine the pomegranate seeds, blueberries, kale, and lemon juice in a blender.

3. Blend until smooth.

4. Strain the mixture through a fine-mesh sieve or cheesecloth into a bowl.

5. Chill before serving.

5. Orange, Carrot, and Spinach Juice

Benefits: Oranges provide vitamin C and antioxidants, carrots offer beta-carotene and fiber, and spinach adds additional fiber and essential nutrients, supporting both blood pressure and blood sugar regulation.

Recipe:

Ingredients:

- 2 oranges, peeled and segmented

- 3 medium carrots, peeled and chopped

- 2 cups fresh spinach leaves

- 1/2 inch piece of fresh ginger, peeled and chopped

Instructions:

1. Wash the spinach leaves thoroughly.

2. Combine the oranges, carrots, spinach, and ginger in a blender.

3. Blend until smooth.

4. Strain the mixture through a fine-mesh sieve or cheesecloth into a bowl.

5. Chill before serving.

Tips for Making and Consuming Juices

1. Use Fresh Ingredients: Always use fresh fruits and vegetables to maximize the nutritional content of your juices.

2. Avoid Added Sugars: Commercially available juices often contain added sugars. Making juices at home allows you to control the ingredients and avoid unnecessary sugars.

3. Consume Immediately: Freshly made juices are best consumed immediately to preserve their nutrient content. If you need to store them, do so in an airtight container in the refrigerator and consume within 24 hours.

4. Balance with Whole Foods: Juices should complement a balanced diet that includes whole fruits and vegetables to ensure adequate fiber intake.

5. Monitor Portion Sizes: Juices can be high in natural sugars and calories, so it's important to consume them in moderation. A serving size of 4-6 ounces is typically sufficient.

6. Consult a Healthcare Provider: If you have pre-existing health conditions or are on medication, consult with a healthcare provider or a registered dietitian before making significant changes to your diet.

Managing blood pressure and blood sugar levels is crucial for maintaining overall health and preventing chronic diseases. Incorporating nutrient-rich juices into your diet can be an effective and enjoyable way to support these health goals. Juices made from spinach, beets, apples, carrots, cucumbers, bitter gourd, and other fruits and vegetables provide a wealth of antioxidants, vitamins, minerals, and bioactive compounds that promote cardiovascular and metabolic health.

The provided recipes offer a variety of delicious and nutritious options that you can easily make at home. Each recipe is designed to maximize the intake of beneficial compounds while being mindful of flavor and nutritional balance. By incorporating these juices into a healthy lifestyle that includes regular physical activity and a balanced diet, you can take significant steps toward managing blood pressure and blood sugar levels, ultimately improving your overall well-being.

Chapter 9

Healthy Basic Nut Milk and Milkshake Recipes

In recent years, the popularity of plant-based diets and dairy alternatives has surged, leading many to explore the world of nut milks and milkshakes. Nut milks offer a nutritious, lactose-free alternative to traditional cow's milk, catering to those with dietary restrictions, lactose intolerance, or those simply looking to add variety to their diet. This comprehensive guide delves into the benefits of nut milks and provides detailed recipes for making various types of nut milks and milkshakes at home. Each recipe is designed to be healthy, delicious, and easy to prepare.

The Benefits of Nut Milks

Nut milks are a great source of essential nutrients, including vitamins, minerals, and healthy fats. Here are some key benefits of incorporating nut milks into your diet:

1. Lactose-Free: Nut milks are a perfect alternative for those who are lactose intolerant or allergic to dairy.

2. Rich in Nutrients: Nut milks often contain vitamins such as E, D, and A, as well as minerals like calcium, magnesium, and potassium.

3. Low in Calories: Many nut milks are lower in calories compared to cow's milk, making them suitable for those looking to manage their weight.

4. Heart Health: Nut milks contain healthy fats that can help improve cholesterol levels and support cardiovascular health.

5. Antioxidant Properties: Nuts are rich in antioxidants, which help protect the body against oxidative stress and inflammation.

Basic Nut Milk Recipes

1. Almond Milk

Benefits: Almond milk is a popular choice due to its mild flavor and versatility. It is rich in vitamin E, which acts as an antioxidant, and provides a good source of calcium and healthy fats.

Recipe:

Ingredients:

- 1 cup raw almonds

- 4 cups water

- 1-2 tablespoons maple syrup or honey (optional, for sweetness)

- 1 teaspoon vanilla extract (optional)

Instructions:

1. Soak the almonds in water overnight or for at least 8 hours. Drain and rinse them.

2. Combine the soaked almonds and 4 cups of water in a blender.

3. Blend on high speed for 2-3 minutes until the almonds are finely ground and the mixture is milky.

4. Strain the mixture through a nut milk bag or a fine-mesh sieve lined with cheesecloth into a bowl, squeezing out as much liquid as possible.

5. If desired, add maple syrup or honey and vanilla extract to the almond milk and stir well.

6. Store the almond milk in an airtight container in the refrigerator for up to 4 days. Shake well before each use.

2. Cashew Milk

Benefits: Cashew milk is creamy and slightly sweet, making it an excellent choice for smoothies and coffee. It is rich in magnesium, which supports muscle and nerve function, and contains healthy monounsaturated fats.

Recipe:

Ingredients:

- 1 cup raw cashews

- 4 cups water

- 1-2 tablespoons agave syrup (optional, for sweetness)

- 1 teaspoon cinnamon (optional)

Instructions:

1. Soak the cashews in water for 4-6 hours. Drain and rinse them.

2. Combine the soaked cashews and 4 cups of water in a blender.

3. Blend on high speed for 2-3 minutes until smooth and creamy.

4. Straining is optional for cashew milk as it blends very smoothly, but if desired, strain through a nut milk bag or fine-mesh sieve lined with cheesecloth.

5. Add agave syrup and cinnamon, if desired, and stir well.

6. Store the cashew milk in an airtight container in the refrigerator for up to 4 days. Shake well before each use.

3. Walnut Milk

Benefits: Walnut milk has a rich, nutty flavor and is packed with omega-3 fatty acids, which are beneficial for brain health. It also contains antioxidants and polyphenols that support heart health.

Recipe:

Ingredients:

- 1 cup raw walnuts

- 4 cups water

- 1-2 tablespoons date syrup (optional, for sweetness)

- 1/2 teaspoon ground nutmeg (optional)

Instructions:

1. Soak the walnuts in water overnight or for at least 8 hours. Drain and rinse them.

2. Combine the soaked walnuts and 4 cups of water in a blender.

3. Blend on high speed for 2-3 minutes until smooth and creamy.

4. Strain the mixture through a nut milk bag or a fine-mesh sieve lined with cheesecloth into a bowl, squeezing out as much liquid as possible.

5. If desired, add date syrup and ground nutmeg, and stir well.

6. Store the walnut milk in an airtight container in the refrigerator for up to 4 days. Shake well before each use.

4. Hazelnut Milk

Benefits: Hazelnut milk has a distinct, sweet, and nutty flavor. It is rich in vitamin E, which supports skin health, and contains healthy fats that promote heart health.

Recipe:

Ingredients:

- 1 cup raw hazelnuts

- 4 cups water

- 1-2 tablespoons coconut sugar (optional, for sweetness)

- 1 teaspoon cocoa powder (optional, for a chocolate flavor)

Instructions:

1. Soak the hazelnuts in water overnight or for at least 8 hours. Drain and rinse them.

2. Combine the soaked hazelnuts and 4 cups of water in a blender.

3. Blend on high speed for 2-3 minutes until smooth and creamy.

4. Strain the mixture through a nut milk bag or a fine-mesh sieve lined with cheesecloth into a bowl, squeezing out as much liquid as possible.

5. If desired, add coconut sugar and cocoa powder, and stir well.

6. Store the hazelnut milk in an airtight container in the refrigerator for up to 4 days. Shake well before each use.

5. Macadamia Nut Milk

Benefits: Macadamia nut milk is incredibly creamy and luxurious, with a subtle buttery flavor. It is high in monounsaturated fats, which support heart health, and contains manganese and thiamine.

Recipe:

Ingredients:

- 1 cup raw macadamia nuts

- 4 cups water

- 1-2 tablespoons maple syrup (optional, for sweetness)

- 1 teaspoon vanilla extract (optional)

Instructions:

1. Soak the macadamia nuts in water for 2-4 hours. Drain and rinse them.

2. Combine the soaked macadamia nuts and 4 cups of water in a blender.

3. Blend on high speed for 2-3 minutes until smooth and creamy.

4. Straining is optional for macadamia nut milk as it blends very smoothly, but if desired, strain through a nut milk bag or fine-mesh sieve lined with cheesecloth.

5. Add maple syrup and vanilla extract, if desired, and stir well.

6. Store the macadamia nut milk in an airtight container in the refrigerator for up to 4 days. Shake well before each use.

Nut Milkshake Recipes

1. Almond and Berry Milkshake

Benefits: This milkshake combines the antioxidant-rich properties of berries with the nutrient-dense almond milk. Berries are low in sugar and high in fiber, making this a healthy treat.

Recipe:

Ingredients:

- 1 cup almond milk (homemade or store-bought)

- 1/2 cup mixed berries (strawberries, blueberries, raspberries)

- 1 banana, frozen

- 1 tablespoon chia seeds (optional, for added fiber)

- 1 tablespoon honey or agave syrup (optional, for sweetness)

Instructions:

1. Combine the almond milk, mixed berries, frozen banana, chia seeds, and honey or agave syrup in a blender.

2. Blend until smooth and creamy.

3. Pour into a glass and serve immediately.

2. Cashew and Mango Milkshake

Benefits: Cashew milk provides a creamy base for this tropical milkshake. Mango is rich in vitamins A and C, and fiber, which aids digestion and supports the immune system.

Recipe:

Ingredients:

- 1 cup cashew milk (homemade or store-bought)

- 1 cup frozen mango chunks

- 1/2 cup Greek yogurt (optional, for added creaminess and protein)

- 1 tablespoon flax seeds (optional, for added fiber)

Instructions:

1. Combine the cashew milk, frozen mango chunks, Greek yogurt, and flax seeds in a blender.

2. Blend until smooth and creamy.

3. Pour into a glass and serve immediately.

3. Walnut and Banana Milkshake

Benefits: Walnut milk provides omega-3 fatty acids and antioxidants, while bananas add natural sweetness, potassium, and fiber. This milkshake is both nutritious and filling.

Recipe:

Ingredients:

- 1 cup walnut milk (homemade or store-bought)

- 1 banana, frozen

- 1 tablespoon almond butter (optional, for added protein)

- 1 teaspoon cinnamon (optional, for flavor)

- 1-2 dates (optional, for added sweetness)

Instructions:

1. Combine the walnut milk, frozen banana, almond butter, cinnamon, and dates in a blender.

2. Blend until smooth and creamy.

3. Pour into a glass and serve immediately.

4. Hazelnut and Chocolate Milkshake

Benefits: This milkshake is a healthier version of a classic chocolate milkshake, using hazelnut milk and cocoa powder. Hazelnut milk provides vitamin E and healthy fats, while cocoa powder adds antioxidants and a rich chocolate flavor.

Recipe:

Ingredients:

- 1 cup hazelnut milk (homemade or store-bought)

- 2 tablespoons unsweetened cocoa powder

- 1 banana, frozen

- 1 tablespoon almond butter (optional, for added creaminess)

- 1-2 tablespoons maple syrup or honey (optional, for sweetness)

Instructions:

1. Combine the hazelnut milk, cocoa powder, frozen banana, almond butter, and maple syrup or honey in a blender.

2. Blend until smooth and creamy.

3. Pour into a glass and serve immediately.

5. Macadamia Nut and Vanilla Milkshake

Benefits: This milkshake features macadamia nut milk, which is creamy and rich, combined with vanilla for a simple yet indulgent treat. Macadamia nuts provide healthy fats and a buttery flavor.

Recipe:

Ingredients:

- 1 cup macadamia nut milk (homemade or store-bought)

- 1 teaspoon vanilla extract

- 1 tablespoon honey or agave syrup (optional, for sweetness)

- 1 cup ice cubes

Instructions:

1. Combine the macadamia nut milk, vanilla extract, honey or agave syrup, and ice cubes in a blender.

2. Blend until smooth and creamy.

3. Pour into a glass and serve immediately.

Nut Milk and Milkshake Variations

1. Pistachio Milk

Benefits: Pistachio milk is unique and flavorful, rich in protein, fiber, and healthy fats. It contains antioxidants and is a good source of B vitamins.

Recipe:

Ingredients:

- 1 cup raw pistachios (shelled)

- 4 cups water

- 1-2 tablespoons agave syrup (optional, for sweetness)

- 1/2 teaspoon cardamom powder (optional, for flavor)

Instructions:

1. Soak the pistachios in water for 4-6 hours. Drain and rinse them.

2. Combine the soaked pistachios and 4 cups of water in a blender.

3. Blend on high speed for 2-3 minutes until smooth and creamy.

4. Strain the mixture through a nut milk bag or fine-mesh sieve lined with cheesecloth into a bowl.

5. If desired, add agave syrup and cardamom powder, and stir well.

6. Store the pistachio milk in an airtight container in the refrigerator for up to 4 days. Shake well before each use.

2. Pistachio and Rose Milkshake

Benefits: This exotic milkshake combines pistachio milk with the delicate flavor of rose water. Pistachios provide protein and fiber, while rose water adds a unique and fragrant twist.

Recipe:

Ingredients:

- 1 cup pistachio milk (homemade or store-bought)

- 1 teaspoon rose water

- 1-2 tablespoons honey (optional, for sweetness)

- 1 cup ice cubes

Instructions:

1. Combine the pistachio milk, rose water, honey, and ice cubes in a blender.

2. Blend until smooth and creamy.

3. Pour into a glass and serve immediately.

3. Brazil Nut Milk

Benefits: Brazil nuts are rich in selenium, a powerful antioxidant that supports thyroid function and immune health. This milk is creamy and slightly nutty in flavor.

Recipe:

Ingredients:

- 1 cup raw Brazil nuts

- 4 cups water

- 1-2 tablespoons maple syrup (optional, for sweetness)

- 1 teaspoon vanilla extract (optional)

Instructions:

1. Soak the Brazil nuts in water for 8-12 hours. Drain and rinse them.

2. Combine the soaked Brazil nuts and 4 cups of water in a blender.

3. Blend on high speed for 2-3 minutes until smooth and creamy.

4. Strain the mixture through a nut milk bag or fine-mesh sieve lined with cheesecloth into a bowl.

5. If desired, add maple syrup and vanilla extract, and stir well.

6. Store the Brazil nut milk in an airtight container in the refrigerator for up to 4 days. Shake well before each use.

4. Brazil Nut and Coconut Milkshake

Benefits: This milkshake combines Brazil nut milk with coconut milk for a creamy and tropical drink. Both ingredients provide healthy fats and antioxidants.

Recipe:

Ingredients:

- 1/2 cup Brazil nut milk (homemade or store-bought)

- 1/2 cup coconut milk

- 1 banana, frozen

- 1 tablespoon coconut flakes (optional, for added texture and flavor)

- 1-2 tablespoons maple syrup (optional, for sweetness)

Instructions:

1. Combine the Brazil nut milk, coconut milk, frozen banana, coconut flakes, and maple syrup in a blender.

2. Blend until smooth and creamy.

3. Pour into a glass and serve immediately.

5. Hemp Seed Milk

Benefits: Hemp seed milk is high in omega-3 and omega-6 fatty acids, which are beneficial for heart health. It is also a good source of protein and contains all essential amino acids.

Recipe:

Ingredients:

- 1 cup hemp seeds

- 4 cups water

- 1-2 tablespoons agave syrup (optional, for sweetness)

- 1 teaspoon vanilla extract (optional)

Instructions:

1. Combine the hemp seeds and 4 cups of water in a blender.

2. Blend on high speed for 2-3 minutes until smooth and creamy.

3. Strain the mixture through a nut milk bag or fine-mesh sieve lined with cheesecloth into a bowl.

4. If desired, add agave syrup and vanilla extract, and stir well.

5. Store the hemp seed milk in an airtight container in the refrigerator for up to 4 days. Shake well before each use.

6. Hemp Seed and Matcha Milkshake

Benefits: This milkshake combines hemp seed milk with matcha powder for a boost of antioxidants and a unique flavor. Matcha also provides a gentle caffeine boost.

Recipe:

Ingredients:

- 1 cup hemp seed milk (homemade or store-bought)

- 1 teaspoon matcha powder

- 1 banana, frozen

- 1 tablespoon chia seeds (optional, for added fiber)

- 1-2 tablespoons honey or agave syrup (optional, for sweetness)

Instructions:

1. Combine the hemp seed milk, matcha powder, frozen banana, chia seeds, and honey or agave syrup in a blender.

2. Blend until smooth and creamy.

3. Pour into a glass and serve immediately.

Tips for Making and Storing Nut Milks and Milkshakes

1. Use Fresh Ingredients: Always use fresh, raw nuts and high-quality ingredients for the best flavor and nutritional content.

2. Soaking Nuts: Soaking nuts not only softens them for blending but also helps reduce phytic acid, which can inhibit nutrient absorption.

3. Sweeteners: Use natural sweeteners like honey, maple syrup, or agave syrup to sweeten your nut milks and milkshakes. Adjust the sweetness to your preference.

4. Straining: While some nut milks blend smoothly and do not require straining, others benefit from being strained through a nut milk bag or cheesecloth for a smoother texture.

5. Storage: Store homemade nut milks in airtight containers in the refrigerator and consume within 3-4 days. Shake well before each use, as separation is natural.

6. Flavor Variations: Experiment with different flavor additions such as vanilla, cinnamon, cocoa powder, or fruit to create unique and delicious variations of nut milks and milkshakes.

Nut milks and milkshakes are versatile, nutritious, and delicious alternatives to traditional dairy products. They cater to a variety of dietary preferences and restrictions while providing essential nutrients and health benefits. By making nut milks and milkshakes at home, you can control the ingredients, avoid additives, and customize flavors to suit your taste. The provided recipes offer a range of options from basic nut milks to indulgent milkshakes, ensuring that there's something for everyone to enjoy. Embrace the world of nut milks and milkshakes and experience the health benefits and delightful flavors they have to offer.

Chapter 10

Soothing Sinus Relief Juices

Sinus congestion and discomfort can be quite bothersome, affecting breathing, sleep, and overall well-being. While medications and remedies are available, natural solutions like sinus relief juices can provide additional support. This guide explores various juices specifically designed to alleviate sinus issues, incorporating ingredients known for their anti-inflammatory, decongestant, and immune-boosting properties. Each recipe aims to soothe sinus discomfort and promote respiratory health.

Understanding Sinus Congestion

Sinus congestion occurs when the nasal passages become inflamed and swollen, often due to allergies, infections, or irritants. Common symptoms include stuffy or runny nose, facial pressure, headaches, and difficulty breathing. Sinus relief juices can help alleviate these symptoms by reducing inflammation, thinning mucus, and supporting the immune system.

Benefits of Sinus Relief Juices

1. Anti-Inflammatory: Ingredients like ginger, turmeric, and citrus fruits possess anti-inflammatory properties that can reduce swelling and discomfort in the sinuses.

2. Decongestant: Spices such as cayenne pepper and horseradish can act as natural decongestants, helping to clear nasal passages and relieve congestion.

3. Vitamin C: Citrus fruits like oranges and lemons are rich in vitamin C, which supports immune function and helps fight off infections.

4. Hydration: Proper hydration is crucial for thinning mucus and keeping nasal passages moist, making juices an excellent way to stay hydrated.

5. Antioxidants: Many fruits and vegetables in these juices are rich in antioxidants, which help reduce inflammation and support overall health.

Sinus Relief Juice Recipes

1. Ginger Turmeric Citrus Juice

Benefits: Ginger and turmeric are potent anti-inflammatory ingredients, while citrus fruits provide vitamin C and a refreshing flavor.

Recipe:

Ingredients:

- 1-inch piece of fresh ginger, peeled

- 1-inch piece of fresh turmeric, peeled (or 1 teaspoon ground turmeric)

- 2 oranges, peeled and segmented

- 1 lemon, peeled and segmented

- 1 tablespoon raw honey (optional, for sweetness)

- 1 cup water or coconut water

Instructions:

1. Place the ginger, turmeric, oranges, lemon, honey (if using), and water/coconut water in a blender.

2. Blend until smooth.

3. Strain the juice through a fine-mesh sieve or cheesecloth to remove pulp.

4. Pour into a glass and serve immediately.

2. Pineapple Mint Eucalyptus Juice

Benefits: Pineapple contains bromelain, an enzyme with anti-inflammatory properties, while mint and eucalyptus provide a cooling sensation and can help clear nasal passages.

Recipe:

Ingredients:

- 1 cup fresh pineapple chunks

- 1/4 cup fresh mint leaves

- 1-2 drops of eucalyptus essential oil (food-grade)

- 1 tablespoon raw honey (optional, for sweetness)

- 1 cup coconut water or plain water

Instructions:

1. Combine the pineapple chunks, mint leaves, eucalyptus oil, honey (if using), and coconut water/plain water in a blender.

2. Blend until smooth.

3. Strain the juice to remove any fibrous bits.

4. Pour into a glass over ice and enjoy immediately.

3. Carrot Apple Ginger Juice

Benefits: Carrots are rich in beta-carotene and antioxidants, while apples add natural sweetness and fiber. Ginger provides anti-inflammatory and immune-boosting benefits.

Recipe:

Ingredients:

- 2 large carrots, peeled and chopped

- 2 apples, cored and chopped

- 1-inch piece of fresh ginger, peeled

- 1/2 lemon, peeled

- 1 cup water

Instructions:

1. Place the carrots, apples, ginger, lemon, and water in a blender.

2. Blend until smooth.

3. Strain the juice if desired or enjoy with the pulp.

4. Pour into a glass and serve chilled or over ice.

4. Beetroot Celery Spinach Juice

Benefits: Beetroots are rich in antioxidants and nitrates, which may help improve blood flow. Celery and spinach add additional vitamins and minerals for overall health.

Recipe:

Ingredients:

- 1 medium-sized beetroot, peeled and chopped

- 2 celery stalks

- 1 cup fresh spinach leaves

- 1/2 cucumber, peeled

- 1/2 lemon, peeled

- 1-inch piece of fresh ginger, peeled

- 1 cup water or coconut water

Instructions:

1. Combine the beetroot, celery, spinach, cucumber, lemon, ginger, and water/coconut water in a blender.

2. Blend until smooth.

3. Strain the juice through a fine-mesh sieve to remove any fibrous bits.

4. Pour into a glass and serve chilled.

5. Spicy Tomato Horseradish Juice

Benefits: Tomatoes are rich in antioxidants and vitamin C, while horseradish acts as a natural decongestant due to its spicy nature.

Recipe:

Ingredients:

- 2 large tomatoes, chopped

- 1/4 cup fresh horseradish, peeled and chopped (adjust to taste)

- 1/2 cucumber, peeled

- 1/2 red bell pepper, seeded and chopped

- 1/2 lemon, peeled

- Dash of cayenne pepper (optional, for extra spiciness)

- 1 cup water or tomato juice

Instructions:

1. Place the tomatoes, horseradish, cucumber, bell pepper, lemon, cayenne pepper (if using), and water/tomato juice in a blender.

2. Blend until smooth.

3. Strain the juice if desired for a smoother texture.

4. Pour into a glass and serve chilled or over ice.

Tips for Making Sinus Relief Juices

1. Fresh Ingredients: Use fresh, organic ingredients whenever possible to maximize nutritional benefits.

2. Peeling and Chopping: For smoother juices, peel and chop fruits and vegetables into smaller pieces before blending.

3. Straining: Strain juices through a fine-mesh sieve or cheesecloth to remove pulp and fiber, if desired.

4. Add Water: If juices are too thick, add water or coconut water to achieve your desired consistency.

5. Temperature: Enjoy juices chilled or over ice for a refreshing experience.

6. Adjust Spice Levels: Some recipes contain spicy ingredients like ginger, horseradish, or cayenne pepper. Adjust these to your taste and tolerance level.

7. Storage: Fresh juices are best consumed immediately for maximum freshness and nutrients. If storing, keep refrigerated and consume within 24-48 hours.

Precautions

- Allergies: Be mindful of any allergies or sensitivities to ingredients used in these recipes.

- Spicy Ingredients: Spicy ingredients like ginger, horseradish, and cayenne pepper may not be suitable for everyone, especially those with sensitive stomachs or acid reflux.

- Consultation: If you have any medical conditions or concerns, consult with a healthcare professional before incorporating new juices into your diet.

Soothing sinus relief juices can be a natural and effective way to alleviate discomfort associated with sinus congestion. By incorporating anti-inflammatory, decongestant, and immune-boosting ingredients into these recipes, you can support respiratory health and promote overall well-being. Whether you prefer the zing of ginger and turmeric or the refreshing coolness of mint and eucalyptus, there's a sinus relief juice for every palate. Enjoy these nutritious and flavorful juices as part of your wellness routine to keep your sinuses clear and your body feeling refreshed.

www.ingramcontent.com/pod-product-compliance
Lightning Source LLC
Chambersburg PA
CBHW081218260726
48653CB00010BB/3679